DATE DUE

Michael C. N̶ ginia Poly-
technic Insti̶ lth-related
topics, inclu̶ and physi-
cal health. I̶ husband,
conducted m̶ ve focused
on nutrition,

MICHAEL C. MOORE
LYNDA J. MOORE

THE COMPLETE HANDBOOK OF HOLISTIC HEALTH

Prentice-Hall, Inc., Englewood Cliffs, New Jersey 07632

Library of Congress Cataloging in Publication Data

Moore, Michael C. (date).
    The complete handbook of holistic health.
    "A Spectrum Book."
    Includes bibliographies and index.
    1. Holistic medicine. 2. Health. 3. Consumer
education. I. Moore, Lynda J., (date).
II. Title
R723.M617 1983   615.5   82-13284
ISBN 0-13-161034-1
ISBN 0-13-161026-0 (pbk.)

This book is available at a special discount when ordered in bulk quantities. Contact Prentice-Hall, Inc., General Publishing Division, Special Sales, Englewood Cliffs, N.J. 07632.

1   2   3   4   5   6   7   8   9   10

ISBN 0-13-161034-1

ISBN 0-13-161026-0 (PBK.)

Cover design by Hal Siegel
Manufacturing buyer: Cathie Lenard

Prentice-Hall International, Inc., *London*
Prentice-Hall of Australia Pty. Limited, *Sydney*
Prentice-Hall Canada Inc., *Toronto*
Prentice-Hall of India Private Limited, *New Delhi*
Prentice-Hall of Japan, Inc., *Tokyo*
Prentice-Hall of Southeast Asia Pte. Ltd., *Singapore*
Whitehall Books Limited, *Wellington, New Zealand*
Editora Prentice-Hall do Brasil Ltda., *Rio de Janeiro*

CONTENTS

PREFACE

When we began this project, we wanted to write a book that would explain the essence of each of the fields of holistic methods we researched. At the same time, we wished to exhibit the benefits as well as the deficiencies of each field. In order to provide enough information for an "understanding" of the fields and enable the reader to see the contradictions, we felt we needed a combination of "impersonal objectivity" and "in-depth subjectivity." We developed categories that would be objective and require us to examine the chosen fields critically. In addition, we intentionally adopted the viewpoints of those in each area so that we could effectively obtain the insights needed to be more than "just informed."

Our search began with a definition of holism so that we could determine how much it had changed, if at all, and if professionals who claimed "holistic" affiliation were, indeed, legitimate in their claims. The theory of holism says that "nature tends to synthesize units into organized wholes." Within holistic medicine this theory translates into the idea that the individual tends to maintain equilibrium within and between its parts. Holism extends to physical, mental, and spiritual aspects of health and to the interrelationship between the individual, the environment, and the world at large.

The notion that the individual has the tendency to maintain balance or harmony is termed *homeostasis* within structured medicine. Holistic practitioners make use of their patient's tendency for equilibrium by encouraging him or her to investigate the sources of disease. Holistic health care is an unfolding process in which professionals and clients share, which results in the healee gaining the knowledge and skill necessary to attain health and well-being.

Since holistic health is the current "trend" in medicine, beware! Currently, there is a great deal of "prostitution" of the word *holistic*, undoubtedly because it appeals to a large number of consumers. There are fields and practitioners that are less than holistic. Holistic healers may be physicians, other health care professionals, or lay persons. Their methods must both treat (find the source of) and prevent disease, although many holistic areas cannot make use of the words *diagnose* and *treat*. Some practitioners in holistic fields prescribe drugs, some fields are composed only of physicians, and other modalities rely strictly upon natural measures for treatment and prevention. This does *not* detract from the particular field, because it is the unique realm of the individual that is important.

Our interest in holistic health has been evolving over the last six years. Both of us were educated as members of the sixties generation, who believed that the individual could make a difference in solving world problems. We both chose teaching as our profession and used positive ways of presenting consumer guidelines to our students so that they could learn to make informed choices in many areas. During the seventies we were fortunate enough to find ourselves doing a study on public health in a rural, mountainous area of southwestern Virginia. We became aware of the reliance of many mountainfolk upon "so-called" folk healers.

During a trip to San Francisco a friend introduced us to a holistic homeopath who was our first contact with "holistic" health. At first we wondered if holism was just another fad. However, as we learned and read more about it, we came to the realization that holistic healing was a modern version of the traditional healers we had met while doing the public health study. During the completion of Mike's work on a Ph.D. in medical sociology, we undertook the project of clarifying holistic health and drawing guidelines to use while teaching.

At first we found that there were almost too many holistic methods to catalogue, and there seemed to be a void when we tried to distinguish between the ones that were fraudulent and those that were legitimate. We began writing professional organizations of alternative medicine, Ralph Nader's Health Research Group, and other consumer-oriented organizations, attempting to find ways to distinguish between the holistic alternatives that were effective and those that were not. We found there were no known ways of making that distinction.

All kinds of "bizarre" methods and healers claimed to be holistic, such as vitamin therapists, pyramidology, graphology, psychic surgery, Laetril therapy, touch encounters, numerology, and astrology. Quite simply, our teaching project became a book because too many of the methods contradicted the meaning of holism. Since we sought to provide an in-depth treatment of several methods or schools of thought, we developed three criteria for deciding whether or not a method should be included:

1. The method had to claim to be holistic, be mentioned in medical journals as holistic, or have an organized profession where its members were trained from a common body of knowledge. This was to avoid the self-styled holistic practitioner who had merely jumped on the latest bandwagon.

2. There had to be some historical evidence for the holistic claim, either in our cultural tradition (for example, homeopathy and naturopathy) or in others (for example, acupuncture and Native American medicine). This is opposed to such purely modern phenomena as biofeedback, for instance, which we include in the historical tradition of meditation. The reason for this criterion was to avoid modern gimmicks and gadgets and to obtain insight into methods that had once worked for our forebears.

3. The holistic method had to be a practice where the consumer could be aware of the healer's method and an active participant in the healing process, which is part of the "modern version" of holistic health. This was in contrast to the consumer as a purely passive recipient who was only needed to pay the bills for a mysterious "cure."

During our screening of many so-called holistic methods, we found fourteen that met all three requirements, and we have devoted a chapter to each. We were not claiming that all the possible types of holistic healing methods were included in this book in an encyclopedic fashion. Instead, we aimed to use these criteria as a first step toward determining those methods that were legitimately holistic.

After the selection we decided to develop a set of consumer criteria that would help people determine if a practitioner was prepared to apply the holistic approach to healing, and we shall review these shortly. Then we took these criteria and constructed a questionnaire, which we mailed to over 500 holistic healers. We received 213 responses. From this information we contacted literally hundreds of holistic health centers and/or clinics and also asked them for information related to the consumer criteria. Finally, we interviewed 307 clients or former clients of holistic healers. With all of this information as a background, we attended workshops in holistic health and read hundreds of books and articles in the fourteen fields.

At first we found ourselves in a maze of conflicting philosophies. Modern medicine is based on the philosophy of *allopathy*, which deals with treating symptoms and providing cures rather than preventing the occurrence of disease. Holistic philosophy encompasses more than physical ailments, it deals with the mind and spirit as well as the body. Whereas allopathy assigns the role of healer to the physician, holism makes healing and preventing an equal partnership between the healer and healee. Finally, one of the major tenets of holism is that once a malady is cured, the fundamental responsibility of *staying* well is that of the healee, not the healer.

From this research a common definition of holistic health emerged. Holistic health is treatment of the whole person, not parts or segments, as is the case in conventional medical practice, where specialization of disease and treatment are the norm. According to the critics of modern medicine, allopaths are more likely to depersonalize medical care through specialization and standardization of the treatment of disease. Holistic practitioners view the entire life of an individual and the interrelationships between illness in the body, on the one hand, and mental, environmental, social, and spiritual states, on the other. Those espousing the holistic philosophy state that the treatment processes of allopathy have led to higher rates of unnecessary surgery, the overprescription of drugs, and rising medical costs for consumers. These facts have served to diminish faith in physicians as "potential gods."

The holistic model maintains that any illness is a combination of a multitude of factors, not germs alone. Additionally, many contemporary healers and scientists believe that a body can immunize itself in order to fight disease and that the individual possesses his or her own healing potential. It follows logically from the perspective of holism, then, that disease is being treated in a narrow manner by orthodox medicine. Consumers are *using* allopathic medicine as a "cure-all" rather than relying upon self-regulating healing potentials.

As consumers of conventional medicine, we think about germs and disease and rely upon doctors and hospitals to provide health and well-being. There are also other problems, more general than germs, that contribute to disease. These include environmental pollution, such basic institutions as family and government, such emotional and social actions as drug abuse and suicide, as well as such mental and spiritual problems as beliefs and essential yearnings. In the midst of the conventional medical model, we feel helpless and do not know where to turn for answers.

Holism emerges as a natural means of determining the multiple contributions we all make to our own health and/or disease in the ways we live and the ideas in which we believe. Holism is a practical philosophy for solving many of the problems that have emerged in the field of health care. As we just mentioned, holistic health holds as its basis the belief that the individual *can do* something about his or her own health. This alternative to conventional medicine combines the most recent advancements in modern science and technology with ancient, natural healing measures that were used in most of the classical civilizations and cultures that have preceded us. Holism fuses ancient and modern ideas with the value of individualism in that each person has an innate healing potential.

Holistic practitioners seek to produce states of "ease" in the body, mind, and spirit of the individual. For example, ask yourself this question: Do all parts of my body feel at ease? If your answer is no, then you may be in a state of *dis-ease*. Furthermore, states of dis-ease are interrelated and can also lead to other symptoms. Not all holistic professionals are certified doctors. Nor are many of them members of the "occult." Since holistic practitioners believe that inherent within each individual is a unique means of healing, they are enthusiastic about your healing potential. They should teach you to recognize your abilities, to use them, and to care about yourself.

Holistic practitioners also suggest ways in which you can take control of your health. You may learn to restructure your diet, eating correct but still enjoyable foods, or taking an hour's nap in the afternoon to provide a relaxed state of mind. You may also learn that your sister "bugs" you with her advice, that you harbor an inner fear of cancer, that you would be happier in another occupation, or that you should put strips of tape on your bathroom tub for safety. According to holistic healers, once you are made aware of the small, everyday factors that damage "a good health posture," you can create changes to rectify them.

The ideal holistic healer personifies the integration of spirit, emotion, mind, and body. This healer encourages a patient to examine his or her environment, which includes life-style, occupation, emotional well-being, social interactions, beliefs, and ecological factors. Any one or all of these can be critical factors affecting the physical health of the individual. This type of self-examination can lead to changes in the way one perceives oneself and others, one's actions, and one's state of health.

According to holistic practitioners, the more actions you take to prevent illness, the less money you will have to spend on curing it. Furthermore, most holistic methods are cheaper than conventional measures. In the long run, holists feel, a holistic approach to health can save you money, just as an investment in a solar energy system saves electricity.

There are many doctors who are holistic healers. In fact, physicians claim that the medicine we experience today was originally holistic. A small segment (400) of the medical profession *is* trying to bridge the gap between conventional medicine and the philosophy of holism. The newly formed American Holistic Medical Association defines holistic health as "a state of being in which an individual's body, mind, emotions, and spirit are in tune with the natural, cosmic, and social environment." Some of these new holistic physicians include drugs and surgery as possible treatments. Many of the holistic professions in this book do not use these except as a last resort. This is their particular bias. However, if you have an appendicitis or a heart attack, you obviously need to consult the appropriate medical specialist.

Our categories are consumer-oriented in that you will be able to judge both the quality of a method's service and the quantity of time and expense. The information we collected in our research is used to provide a *definition* of each healing modality, a characterization of the *type of healing* utilized by each group of healers, and a *description of the healing method* practiced in each instance. These three consumer criteria are intended to give you, the reader, a basic idea of what you would be getting into if you choose to utilize holistic services. In this way you will be able to seek them out knowing what to expect. We also include information on the *diseases* that are *treated* by specific practitioners as well as the approximate *duration of their treatments*. There will usually be a wide array of specific maladies treated by each practitioner. A *cost range* of services for each field is also included as a guide by which the informed consumer can decide whether it is economically feasible to visit a practitioner.

Furthermore, in keeping with the basic holistic tenet that you possess the innate potential to heal or regulate yourself, we provide a section on the *personal responsibilities* that consumers will be expected to assume in conjunction with each method of healing. By assuming these responsibilities and practicing them on a daily basis, you will not only enhance a particular method or technique, but you will learn to prevent symptoms from reoccurring. Practitioners assert that they seek to change your life-style from one oriented toward dis-ease to one focused on ease and personal well-being. There is a list of *informational organizations* for each field so that you can write for referrals, educational materials, or services.

Finally, we point out where each method is *consistent* with the principles of holism outlined in this introduction. We also take the liberty of discussing their *inconsistencies* in order to provide consumers with a list of the strengths and weaknesses of each healing field we explore in our research. These criteria do not necessarily follow one another. They are only numbered for convenience. In other words, inconsistency 1 is not meant to be the opposite of consistency 1 and vice versa. Further, at times the inconsistencies with the holistic philosophy may be extended to include contradictions within the field being discussed. We include a large number of *resources* for each holistic measure. This will help you obtain reading material in each field.

Contained in the book are a wide array of holistic practitioners ranging from music therapists to herbalists and naturopaths, to chiropractors and nutritionists. We do not advocate these as the only fields within holism. There are others that we have omitted for the reasons described. Remember, we have tried to select the methods you are likely to encounter in holistic healing centers and practices around the country, not just in one particular area.

After completing this book, we found that what we started out viewing as alternatives to modern medicine are now becoming more accepted as "legitimate" healing practices. We make note of this with the knowledge that each of us must decide upon his or her own combination of healing methods in order to attain a higher state of well-being. We hope we have furnished you with some answers to your basic questions about holistic health methods. You can be your own judge, since ultimately you are responsible for your own well-being.

This book, we hope, will give readers an understanding of holistic methods, insight into individual responsibility for health, some strategies for promoting health, and factual reporting on the inadequacies of various holistic health fields being used today. Finally, we wish to facilitate for the reader the transition from specialized medical care to whole-person medical care. We deeply appreciate the practitioners and their former clients for aiding our investigation of these holistic methods. Without their sincere wish for our enlightenment, this work would not be possible.

Lastly, we must thank Diane Thorup for services at the typewriter, the Whites for a warm fire, canasta, and snacks; and Kit Calhoun-Laman, a counterpart, for her own labor of love and friendship.

Mike and Lynda Moore offer educational and counseling services in all aspects of holistic health. Those who are interested in learning more about holistic health, or any of its various aspects, may contact them through: Ms. Carol Lundberg, M.H.A., Health Quest, Inc., P.O. Box 384, Lake Worth, Florida 33460.

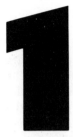

NUTRITIONAL THERAPY

Definition

Nutritional therapy is one of the most battle-ridden fields within holistic health. This is primarily due to the fact that many self-styled "experts" have made nutrition their "home." The growth of the health food industry has also contributed to a large subculture centered around the words *natural* and *organic*. For the consumer this field is highly representative of the confusing maze of therapies known as holistic. Holistic nutritional therapists believe that "you are what you eat, where you eat, with whom you eat, and what you see and hear while eating, what you think about or feel while eating, and—oh yes—everything else that ever happens to you."*

*From the book *Inner Balance: The Power of Holistic Healing* by Elliott M. Goldwag, ed. © 1979 by Elliott M. Goldwag. Published by Prentice-Hall, Inc., Englewood Cliffs, New Jersey, 07632.

Nutrition is a science concerned with the use of foods for body function. Its focus includes the chemical and biological processes associated with maintaining body function for the individual. The science is based in organic chemistry but its scope is also the internal and external interactions between foods and environment. Nutrition, then, is composed of the processes of assimilation, growth, conversion, and excretion in living organisms. Environmental concerns are food supplies, safety, education, and social patterns linked to foods.

Within nutritional science is a branch of hygiene known as *dietetics*. *Dietitians* treat individuals or groups through diet. They are most often employed by schools, hospitals, and other institutions for the purpose of designing special diets or meals for a large number of people. However, they also design "normal" diets. Dietitians are part of the health network in that they are well versed in hygiene and trained in the practical application of dietetics to health and dis-ease.

Nutritionists, on the other hand, specialize in the problems and processes of nutrition. Strictly speaking, nutritionists are more theoretically oriented in that they have not been trained in the practical applications of diet, as dietitians have. Whereas both nutritionists and dietitians have many of the same courses in their curriculum, the American Dietetic Association establishes criteria and administers the national exam by which professionals become registered (or licensed) dietitians. According to a nutritionist in one university, those with a minimum of a B.S. in nutrition are nutritionists, while either nutritionists or those trained in dietetics can become registered dietitians if they qualify by taking a specialized core of courses that apply sound dietary principles to health. Nutritional therapists might be either nutritionists or dietitians. Many experts feel that the use of the terms *nutritional therapist* and *diet therapist* is ambiguous and recommend that consumers investigate the credentials of all of those claiming that status. This division between dietitians and nutritionists is irrelevant, for both are *educators* and both are well informed in the scientific processes and individual considerations within nutrition. In fact, the official distinctions between them become blurred when they are viewed in this manner.

Nutritional therapists who subscribe to holistic beliefs, then, must also possess credentials in the field. Consequently, many nutritional "consultants" currently within holism have made themselves such and are not legitimate nutritional therapists. Holistic nutritional therapists advocate a moderate position between the scientific world and the world of health food faddists. For example, they do not usually recommend weight reduction clinics or medical centers to control weight. Instead, they prefer to teach clients that weight problems can be resolved by ingesting the proper proportions and combinations of foods, engaging in physical exercise, and altering eating patterns.

Therapists of holistic nutrition are caught between faddists and scientists in other ways. The FDA reports that there is little difference between processed and refined foods and organic foods and that pesticides and residual limits are low enough to protect consumers (HEW publication no. 79–2108, FDA). Holistic therapists in this field point out that the biochemical balance within the body can be altered by chemicals, regardless of the FDA reports. For example, Dr. P. M. Newberne of MIT says, "Pesticides, especially the chlorinated hydrocarbons along with chlorinated dibenzofurans, are widespread in our environment and result in pathologic changes in animals" (1980). With evidence such as this, one nutritionist told us, many therapists prefer that their clients consume foods in their most natural state (little cooking) and that all foods be washed thoroughly before they are prepared or eaten.

Likewise, legitimate nutritional therapists only rarely suggest that the consumer rely upon supplements. They are of the belief that essential vitamin and mineral nutrients can be attained through foods. Recommended daily allowances (RDA's) are not requirements for every individual. They are, instead, flexible standards. A varied diet, the experts agree, assures consumers of receiving all that is needed to maintain body functioning. Some holistic therapists make use of fasting for short periods of time at the beginning of their treatment. But since they assert that "starvation" can reduce lean body tissue, fasting is supplemented with such foods as dry milk, fish, or even cottage cheese. Further, they suggest their clients exercise caution and maintain supervision while fasting.

Much can be said about the cooking of foods, and instruction about food preparation is an integral aspect of holistic nutritional therapy. Practitioners point out that it makes sense that heat destroys the natural life-giving qualities within foods. If even more of the life is destroyed when cooking, it is reasoned, there is little food value remaining by the time it is eaten. Drying, roasting, frying, or boiling all cause the destruction of important vitamins and trace elements within foods. From a nutritional perspective, overcooking foods and eating the incorrect amounts and combinations of foods are the major causes of most nutritionally oriented dis-eases in the body. Some practitioners also assert that foods from your own area are best for the body: local vegetable and fruit stands supposedly have fresher foods than products shipped to the grocery store.

One way to prevent dis-ease, according to nutritional therapists, is to teach clients the scientific facts about nutrition, alter eating patterns, and design individual diets that provide both variety and nutrients. Since many nutritional dis-eases are caused by eating inadequately, nutritional therapists use several methods to analyze the kinds and combinations of foods taken into the body on a daily and a weekly basis. After analysis a diet is then designed based upon the unique balance and needs of each body so that the internal environment of the client promotes balance.

Throughout the reeducation process provided by holistic nutritionists, one learns to choose a variety of foods, to cook foods in a manner that prevents the loss of valuable nutrients, and to plan menus suitable to the individual's needs and tastes. Additionally, consumers are taught that there are no "good" or "bad" foods but only "correct and incorrect" combinations and proportions of foods. The daily environment of the client is also discussed during educational sessions.

Many nutritionists refer to water as being the "forgotten element." Water is a fundamental property of existence and therefore a vital component in nutritional education. Water performs a variety of functions in our bodies. It regulates body temperature, mixes with food substances, lubricates, serves as a solvent, and participates in digestion and absorption processes. For these reasons, nutritional education incorporates the study of planning balanced, individual diets, discussions of adequate water intake, cooking and shopping practices, and exercise. However, in most holistic settings, we found that exercise does not receive as much attention as the other components of nutritional education.

Although there was little coverage of the event, in 1977 the Senate Select Committee on Nutrition and Human Needs recommended ten major nutritional goals for the public. The established goals can be used as guides to the foods that enhance our health. Additionally, by adhering to their recommendations, Americans can drastically change their eating habits. The committee suggested that we

1. Increase carbohydrate consumption to account for 55 to 60 percent of the energy (caloric) intake.
2. Reduce overall fat consumption from approximately 40 to 30 percent of energy intake.
3. Reduce saturated fat consumption to account for about 10 percent of total energy intake; and balance that with polyunsaturated and monounsaturated fats, which should account for about 10 percent of energy intake each.
4. Reduce cholesterol consumption to about 300 milligrams a day.
5. Reduce sugar consumption by about 40 percent to account for about 15 percent of total energy intake.
6. Reduce salt consumption by about 50 to 85 percent to approximately 3 grams a day
7. Increase consumption of fruits, vegetables, and whole grains.
8. Decrease consumption of meat and increase consumption of poultry and fish.
9. Decrease consumption of foods high in fat, and partially substitute polyunsaturated fat for saturated fat.
10. Substitute nonfat milk for whole milk.

Interestingly enough, Irving Wallace, Amy Wallace, and David Wallechinsky in *Parade* magazine recently reported on the repercussions of these nutritional guidelines by "certain business lobbies." The authors allege that certain food industries (meat, eggs, sugar, canning, dairy, and grain) complained about being slighted by the Senate Committee. The authors go on to say that the most severe strike against the committee's recommendations came from the AMA, which said that there was "no proof that diet is related to disease."*

Consequently, the suggestions made by the committee have been somewhat altered. In summary, the *new* recommendations urge lean meats with poultry and fish, limiting refined and processed sugars, and higher consumption of salt and eggs. Regardless of the accusations made by lobbyists and the AMA, the holistic nutritional consultants whom we interviewed believe that the dietary goals for the United States, as stated by the committee in 1977, are excellent guidelines for conscientious consumers to follow. However, they further explain that dietary goals should be used in combination with recommended daily allowances because they (the RDA's) represent what is a *nutritionally adequate* diet, whereas the goals do not.

This controversy is a logical by-product of economic forces in our society. Another case in point is the nutritional/economic controversy over the nutrient value of white bread, one of the staples of the American diet. White bread is often challenged by consumers advocating a return to natural foods in the form of whole wheat bread. In this instance, there is evidence to support their claim. Borenstein (1980: 499), an academic nutritionist, points out that the most significant vitamin losses in processing occur while whole wheat is milled to produce white flour. He asserts that more than 75 percent of the vital nutrients of the flour are separated out. The consumer, in all of these conflicts between the vested interests of the food industry and the holistic nutritional concern for health and safety, is left with a feeling of uncertainty over which "guidelines" to choose.

According to Professor A. E. Axelrod, a biochemist, there is an association between nutritional deficiencies and immune response in experimental animals (1980: 588). There are difficulties in generalizing these results to humans. Conflicts, then, do arise over the applicability of these findings. However, since we believe that these correlations are important, two should be included as "food for thought." One is that the requirements of amino acids and vitamin B complex are commonly recognized by nutritional biochemists as being significantly related to an immune response on the part of the body. The other is that under certain conditions, a decreased intake of protein has actually led to an increased

*"Significa," *Parade*, June 7, 1981.

immune response. The latter finding most certainly supports the recommendation of holistic nutritionists to decrease the consumption of red meats and whole grains.

There is a category of healers within structured medicine called *orthomolecular physicians*, who rely primarily upon nutrition and vitamins as means for treatment of dis-ease. Most of these doctors treat their clients with megavitamin therapy. Holistic practitioners and physicians state that orthomolecular medicine will be an important field in the future of the holistic health movement. However, since we could find no historical precedent for this school of thought, we have purposely left these therapists out of our discussion on nutrition. Although many dis-eases are related to vitamins and minerals, we feel that megavitamins are not the best means for treatment or prevention of dis-ease.

There are many holistic professionals who disagree on the safety of vitamins, especially when prescribed in large doses. It is their belief that large amounts of *any* substance decrease the body's efficiency to obtain them from daily consumption. Consequently, "large doses of these elements weaken the body's ability to extract these same elements from food and eventually a dependency is created" (Kaslof, 1978). Be sure to check into all the details of vitamin therapy. Too much of one substance can be as dangerous as too little.

In addition, nutritionists assert that vitamins that are labeled as being derived from "natural sources" are often synthetic. The controversy between nutritionists and health food faddists is intense. According to nutritionists, so-called health food stores which supply the consumer with many "organic" and "natural" foods often falsely promote substances, especially vitamins and minerals. The food and advertising industries capitalize upon consumer concern for safe, chemical-free foods. Consequently, millions of dollars have been poured into relabeling efforts, advertising, and, in many cases, outright fraud. For example, one store in California could not determine the "natural sources" from which a particular vitamin was derived. This manager found that labeling vitamins natural not only increased the price but also that the label did not necessarily mean the food came from a "natural" source. The manager removed all natural vitamin supplements from the store and requested that customers buy them from a pharmacy. (FDA Consumer, July–August, 1978.)

The battle between "health" foods and foods that compose the customary American diet will not end in the near future. Consumers, then, must not be fooled by the words *natural*, *organic*, or *health foods* because they are employed interchangeably by food industries. There are few "facts" that can be attributed to health foods being more beneficial than processed foods. And, because most fad foods and diets do not make *direct* claims that can be proven false, consumers must be especially cautious about spending extra money to purchase health foods. Nutritional therapy is plagued by a multitude of self-styled "experts," who are not trained in the scientific principles of nutrition or dietetics. These experts usually promote nutrition as a cure for disease. Many are also of the belief that vitamins and minerals can cure or prevent disease.

Nutritional Faddists

1. Support claims with pamphlets containing indirect evidence.
2. Claim or suggest cures and preventions through natural foods or supplements.
3. Use the words *organic, health* and *natural* interchangeably.
4. Suggest paying more money for natural substances, although they may have no personal assurance that the substance is actually natural.

As many holistic nutritionists point out, proponents of the health food industry also have legitimate concerns regarding chemical additives and fertilizers. But, they assert, this concern has been generalized so that it embraces all food substances available to the consumer. Frankly, the composition of federal regulations tends to support such claims. While Bernard Oser (1980: 506–518) tells us that scientists believe that natural foods are also complex mixtures of chemicals that can even be toxic in excessive dosage, he describes the Federal Environmental Pesticide Control Act as being responsible for admitting pesticides as an "economic poison" under the law. The Food, Drug and Cosmetic Act, on the other hand, regulates additives, the largest proportion of which are flavoring agents. Though tests of additives are performed on animals, there are no specific experimental conditions for measuring the carcinogenic potential of them. Thus, there is not a legal concept of an additive having absolutely no carcinogen. It is obvious, therefore, that neither scientists nor the government have a "real" idea of the effects of additives on health. That is why holistic nutritionists suggest caution in consuming processed foods.

Nutritional therapists are a key factor in treating one of the most common dis-eases of our planet: obesity. So-called "medical centers" and diet fads prey upon the American public with their programs for weight reduction. Holistic nutritionists point out that the types of measures employed by the majority of such places are seldom effective in rectifying weight problems. They explain that treatments such as harmone shots and/or specific dieting practices produce an imbalance in the body. Even though one may lose some weight, it is usually gained back. In fact, according to therapists, clients are often persuaded to join the "center," pay for treatment in advance, and sign a contract before finding out the actual content of their programs.

Holistic nutritionists seek to restructure diet practices without sacrificing one's taste for food or a balanced, nutritionally sound diet. They point out that problems of overindulgence are commonly associated with an individual's eating patterns. Nutritionists further contend that the client must be self motivated, have reinforcement from family and friends and engage in some sort of energy output to lose weight permanently. Practitioners seek to restructure dietary habits so that an individual loses weight and preserves health. The major focus of this therapy is education that emphasizes altered beliefs about and patterns associated with eating.

Unfortunately, physicians who have felt the need to incorporate nutritional therapy into their practice report that patients do not respond well to counseling by a nutritionist. Nutritional therapists who work with physicians are often resented by patients. Consequently, some innovative and concerned physicians have had to cut this aspect of their care or risk losing some "fat fees."

Within most all holistic practices, nutrition is considered one of the most important aspects in preventing dis-ease because it is an essential element for furthering life. Holistic nutritional therapists are educators who teach that in order for the body to adapt to the constant change one experiences, an internal and external balancing must take place. Internal balancing is created by healthy eating habits, water consumption and body awareness. External change is focused on energy exchange, cooking and shopping practices, and restructured eating patterns. Furthermore, the multitude of interactions between these and the individual is important. "Healing" is not the "duty" of a nutritionist, but their therapy is an excellent supplement to any health care practice. Therapy from a holistic nutritional therapist is accomplished through dietary analysis, counseling, recommended dietary change, education, and cooperation from the client.

Type of Healing

Since nutritional therapists are primarily educators, they do not consider themselves to be healers. Simply put, most nutritionists are of the belief that the general public is not aware of the importance of water intake, the effects overcooking has on foods' life-giving properties, the adequate amounts and combinations of foods to eat, their overindulgence in junk foods containing "empty" calories, and the problems associated with all of these working in combination. Consequently, this profession has taken upon itself the task of informing the public about these factors in addition to advocating their services to rectify problems.

Nutritional therapists are primarily concerned with deficiency dis-eases, dis-eases related to emotional health and dis-eases related to excessive amounts of food in the system. Most therapists report that these types of dis-eases can be corrected with individualized dietary and environmental changes. (In many cases vitamin and mineral supplements are also recommended.) Likewise, nutritionists state that other environmental factors, such as psychological state, pollution, and job satisfaction, can also be important in solving nutritional problems.

The individual, often unaware of the great numbers of factors influencing well-being, must establish a procedure for a wide array of conditions. Holistic therapists contend that all components of the individual—spiritual, mental, physical, and environmental—have an effect on food absorption and body functioning. To rectify the lack of individual knowledge, client counseling is an intricate part of nutritional therapy. Sessions can be individual or in groups and concentrate upon pinpointing deleterious eating patterns as well as discussing dietary problems and answering questions about the therapy. Furthermore, this type of experience provides the client with self-help methods in that throughout the sessions an individualized health maintenance program is continually examined and changed to meet specific needs. It is hoped that enlightened clients can then choose among a multitude of procedures to solve a problem, prevent nutritional deficiences and excesses, and adapt to changing situations.

Description of Healing Method

As a client, one should expect a lengthy first visit. The "examination" includes discussion of many aspects of health. This means that dietary intake, physical activity, psychological concerns, spiritual questions, and environmental factors are explored by the holistic nutritionist. Some therapists provide a very general physical examination and some therapists require tests on hair, urine, blood, and dietary (chemical) balance (see the following box). Many practitioners are able to make these tests within the office setting, but a few suggest specific laboratories or hospital settings for this procedure. Finally, a general counseling session is held wherein "fact sheets" about nutrition are given to the client, discussion of dis-ease prevention takes place, and suggestions for minor dietary changes are recommended.

Methods Used by Nutritionists for Dietary Analysis

Anthropometric—Document weight, height, skinfold thickness, etc.

Clinical—Visible signs, such as dry hair, pale skin, dermatitis, etc.

Biochemical—Blood, urine, stool, hair analysis

Dietary—Survey of food intake

During the second visit attention will be given to the test results. One usually talks with the physician or directing professional, who explains the meaning of the tests and how they relate to your specific dis-ease. In most cases, clients also consult with a nutritional counselor. During your time spent with the counselor, dietary and life-style patterns are designed by client and practitioner based on the complete information gathered during the first visit. It is crucial here to point out that physicians who have hired a nutritional counselor and have included him or her in the medical practice place faith in the ability of the nutritionist to design and recommend dietary changes. Compliance with "prescribed" treatment given by the nutritionist is equally important to the physician.

Subsequent visitations revolve around counseling, reorganizing diet, and nutritional education. One of the major problems facing nutritionists is how to teach consumers the simplest way to ensure they are planning a menu containing the essential ingredients for optimal body functioning. Most nutritionists teach clients to choose a variety of foods from the four basic food groups: milk, meat, vegetables and fruits, bread and cereals. Nutritionists also suggest other means (see the following box). Each of the "accepted" ways of evaluating nutritional intake has limitations, which suggests that a thorough understanding of food's relationship to health is complicated. In some nutritional practices, physical exercise and relaxation measures are also explained. Clients practice stress reduction measures, plan meals, and receive instruction on how to maintain an adequate diet when therapy is no longer required.

Nutritional Evaluation Tools for Consumer Use

Tool	How It Works
4 Basic Food Groups	Consumer chooses 4 servings from each group.
Exchange Lists	Six lists of foods that emphasize energy: nutrient content.
Nutritional Labeling	Product labels presenting the RDA's for the average eighteen-year-old male.
Index of Nutritional Quality (INQ)	Individualizes nutrient needs and food's contribution to total energy intake.
Nutrition Scoreboard	Foods are given points for nutrient value.

Some nutritional therapists include fasting in their counseling. They point out that fasting eliminates poisons in the body. (Therapists are careful to warn clients about employing fasting procedures without the aid of a qualified nutritional consultant.) As mentioned earlier, most fasts are supplemented with some sort of food consumption. The fasting process can last from two to five days, depending upon the professional.

Holistic nutritional therapists will most likely ask one to alter various life-style patterns they consider to be dangerous for proper body functioning. Not every person will require drastic changes, but, according to these professionals, body, mind, spirit, and environment must be considered in order to assure the prevention of dis-ease. The fact that professionals and physicians who adhere to the holistic philosophy incorporate nutritional guidance into their specific healing modality has "proven" the dramatic relevance of food and health.

Diseases Treated

Many dis-eases that may be linked to nutrition are as yet "officially" undiscovered simply because past research has been limited or inconclusive due to small sample size and animal experiments. Some of the dis-eases aided by nutritional therapists are heart disease, anemia, cancer, hypotension and hypertension, hyperactivity, constipation, hypoglycemia, hyperglycemia, kidney stones and kidney disease, tooth decay, shingles, herpes, schizophrenia, varicose veins, prostate problems, goiter, diabetes, depression, asthma, arteriosclerosis, obesity, scurvy, rickets, hemorrhoids, ulcers, gout, allergies, and many other deficiency (such as anorexia nervosa) and over sufficiency dis-eases related to vitamins and minerals. Nutritional therapy is especially effective for allergies, arthritis, and heart disease.

Duration of Treatment

Most nutritional professionals require a minimum of three office visits but prefer that clients acquire knowledge about a wide variety of facts relating to nutrition. A much longer period may be necessary in order to implement these facts into daily life. Holistic therapy sessions average two hours and can last up to six months. Previous clients indicate that therapy usually takes three months so that nutritional recommendations can be evaluated and altered if needed. During much of this time the client determines his or her own needs and tastes for nutritional health.

The effects of nutritional changes are apparent in two to three days. In some cases, therapeutic effects take as long as three weeks. Nutritional alternatives are often permanent ones, so problems do not recur.

Cost Range

The cost will vary depending upon whether you are going to a clinic, professional nutritionist, physician, workshop, or a combination of these.

Physician—$20–$30 per visit.

Nutritionist—$12–$25 per visit (unless included with physician)

Follow-up counseling—$10–$25

Laboratory tests—$105–$250 (per series including hair, blood, urine, and chemical analysis)

$35–$70 per test

One-week clinic—$250 and up (may or may not include room and board)

Two-week clinic—$350 and up (may or may not include room and board)

Individual workshops—$7.50–$15 per educational or self-help course

Personal Responsibilities

Initially, you will be expected to monitor food intake, which may mean you will have to make a list of all foods eaten for a specific period of time. Further monitoring is needed to assemble the body's reactions to foods. Along these lines, clients must assume responsibility for including nourishment recommendations into regular eating habits. This will require shopping outside the supermarket, preparing foods in a way that vital nutrients are not destroyed, and balancing the correct combinations and proportions of food.

Since no definitive guidelines for licensure have been established for nutritionists, consumers should make sure the nutritional therapist they wish to consult falls into one of the following categories: (1) He or she has attained a minimum of a B.S. in the field of nutrition, preferably an M.S. or a Ph.D., and is active in professional associations; (2) He or she is a licensed dietitian who may prescribe nutritional therapy. This category can include a wide array of different health professionals, including nutritionists, biochemists, those with an M.S. in public health, in addition to dietitians and physicians. Perhaps the best guideline we can provide for you for choosing a practitioner in this field is to call your local chapter of the American Dietetics Association and/or other nutritional associations or the department of dietetics or nutrition in a local university, then ask about the credibility of the nutritional therapist you wish to consult.

In some cases, it is the consumer's charge to obtain hair, urine, blood, and chemical testing. Should you decide to make use of nutritional therapy, it would be to your advantage to shop around for prices. A public health clinic is often the least expensive and faster.

This can also speed up treatment, since you will have the tests for the initial visitation.

You must be extremely cautious about nutritional practitioners. Because many self-styled nutritional experts have found a place under the rubric of holistic health, be sure to check into the credentials of any dietary counselor. Nutrition quackery can kill as well as cure. Do not be fooled by the persuasive techniques of health food faddists or those advertising "surefire" ways to lose weight. Stand back and evaluate the attributes and limitations of "natural" vitamins or "organic" foods before deciding to purchase one of these products. One way to do this is to ask yourself this question: Why does something cost more if it does not require processing? Before joining a "medical center" that specializes in nutritional therapy, find out exactly what means are put to use to help you lose weight, then sign the contract or make payment if you wish.

Informational Organizations

International Academy of Biological Medicine, Inc.
PO Box 31313
Phoenix, AZ 85046

American Academy of Medical Preventics
11211 Cararillo Street
North Hollywood, CA 91602

International College of Applied Nutrition
PO Box 386
La Harbra, CA 90631

Nutrition Education Center, Inc.
PO Box 303
Oyster Bay, NY 11771

Consistencies

1. Although there is uncertainty concerning the scientific information available on the effectiveness of nutritional therapy, practitioners report that many are "cured" of a wide range of illnesses by nutrition. This could be due to the association between the self-regulating immune system of the body and nutrients.

2. Clients and therapists work together gathering information, planning an individualized health program, and altering recommendations no longer suitable. The client experiences increased awareness of bodily processes and nutrient interactions that facilitate therapy.

3. Educational seminars and counseling focus on self-help and health maintenance through nutrition, so that the consumer is able to apply the information learned at home. Relaxation measures are also included in some settings so that consumers are able to deal more effectively with environmental stressors related to eating patterns.

4. Physical exercise is recommended by holistic nutritionists to facilitate energy exchange. Therapists believe that exercise is an additional measure that promotes health and well-being.

5. Because of intensive educational training, previous clients report they are better able to detect the onset of nutritionally oriented dis-eases. Therapists feel that this is a valuable tool enabling the consumer to prevent dis-ease.

Inconsistencies

1. Even though the field of nutrition is growing by leaps and bounds, there are still fewer nutritionists than other professionals who make use of nutritional therapy within other fields. This seems to contradict the claim that nutritional science should be integrated into structured medicine. It appears that professionals have not been able to convince orthodox medicine of its qualities that prevent an "integrated approach to health." Nutritionists seem relatively inactive as a group to influence food industries. It is also likely that were the AMA to back up claims made by nutritionists, change would currently be taking place.

2. This field is much more expensive than most other holistic measures because of the testing required. Numbers and prices of laboratory tests vary considerably, and certain tests are not always needed. Retesting is usually suggested by these therapists, which doubles the cost to consumers.

3. Vitamin and mineral dosage is a controversy that separates nutritionists and physicians. This conflict seems to be a moot point, since both purport that vitamins and minerals should be prescribed based upon individual circumstances.

4. One reason for the battle-ridden nature of this field, perhaps, is the different belief systems of the various parties concerning diet and nutrition. We recommend that the consumer work to practice adequate nutrition, however the definition of this term may change, as a vital ingredient of health for the whole person.

Sources to Read

Adams, Ruth. *Eating in Eden: The Nutritional Superiority of "Primitive" Foods.* Emmaus, PA: Rodale Press, 1976.

Airola, Paavo O. *Are You Confused?* Phoenix, AZ: Health Plus, 1971.

——. *How to Get Well.* Phoenix, AZ: Health Plus, 1974.

Ardell, Donald B., ed. *High-Level Wellness: An Alternative to Doctors, Drugs, and Disease.* Emmaus, PA: Rodale Press, 1977.

Axelrod, A. E. "Nutrition in Relation to Immunity," *Modern Nutrition in Health and Disease,* ed. Robert Goodhart and Maurice Shils. Philadelphia: Lea and Febiger, 1980.

Ballentine, Rudolph, M.D. *Diet and Nutrition.* Honesdale, PA: Himalayan International Institute of Yoga Science and Philosophy, 1978.

Beiler, Henry G. *Food Is Your Best Medicine.* New York: Random House, 1965.

Bezanson, David P. *Holistic Health.* Albuquerque, NM: Sun Publishing, 1977.

Bircher-Brenner, M. *Eating Your Way to Health.* Baltimore: Penguin, 1973.

Borenstein, Benjamin. "Effect of Processing on the Nutritional Values of Foods," in *Modern Nutrition in Health and Disease.* ed. Robert Goodhart and Maurice Shils. Philadelphia, PA: Lea and Febiger, 1980.

Bruch, H. *Eating Disorders.* New York: Basic Books, 1973.

Carque, Otto. *Vital Facts about Foods: A Guide to Health and Longevity.* New Canaan, CT: Keats, 1975.

Cheraskin, Emanuel, M.D., and **Ringsdorf, W., M.D.** *Predictive Medicine.* Mountain View, CA: Pacific Press Publishing Association, 1973.

Colimore, Benjamin and **Colimore, Sarah.** *Nutrition and Your Body.* Los Angeles: Phoenix House, 1974.

Elwood, Catharyn. *Feel Like a Million.* New York: Pocket Books, 1973.

Gammon, Margaret. *The Normal Diet.* Virginia Beach, VA: ARE Press, 1976.

General Foods Corporation. *Today's Food Additives.* White Plains, NY: General Foods Corporation, 1976.

Goldwag, William, M.D. "Self-Regulation Through Nutrition," in *Inner Balance: The Power of Holistic Healing,* ed. Elliott M. Goldwag. Englewood Cliffs, NJ: Prentice-Hall, 1979.

Gunderson, Eric, and **Rache, R.** *Life Stress and Illness.* Springfield, IL: Charles C. Thomas, 1974.

Kadans, Joseph M. *Encyclopedia of Fruits, Vegetables, Nuts and Seeds for Healthful Living.* Los Angeles, CA: Prentice-Hall, 1973.

Kaslof, Leslie J. *Wholistic Dimensions in Healing.* Garden City, NY: Doubleday, 1978.

Keyes, Ken, Jr. *Loving Your Body.* Berkeley, CA: Living Love Center, 1974.

Kirchmann, J.D., ed. *Nutrition Almanac.* New York: McGraw-Hill, 1975.

Kloss, Jethro. *Back to Eden.* Santa Barbara, CA: Woodbridge Press, 1975.

Kreutler, Patricia A., Ph.D. *Nutrition in Perspective.* Englewood Cliffs, NJ: Prentice-Hall, 1980.

Longgood, William. *Poisons in Your Food.* New York: Pyramid, 1969.

Null, Gary, and **Null, S.** *Complete Handbook of Nutrition.* New York: Dell, 1973.

Oser, Bernard. "Chemical Additives in Foods," in *Modern Nutrition in Health and Disease,* ed. Goodhart and Shils. Philadelphia: Lea and Febiiger, 1973.

Pelstring, Linda, and **Hauck, J. A.** *Food to Improve Your Health: A Complete Guide to Over Three Hundred Foods for One Hundred One Common Ailments.* New York: Walker, 1974.

Popenoe, Chris, comp. *Wellness.* Washington, DC: Y.E.S. Publishing, 1977.

Reilly, Harold J., and **Brod, R. H.** *Edgar Cayce Handbook for Health Through Drugless Therapy.* New York: Macmillan, 1975.

Reuben, David. *Everything You Always Wanted to Know about Nutrition.* New York: Simon and Schuster, 1978.

Ridakem, Herine U. *Complete Book of Minerals for Health.* Emmaus, PA: Rodale Press, 1972.

Robbins, William. *American Food Scandal.* New York: William Morrow, 1974.

Taub, Harold. *Keeping Healthy in a Polluted World.* New York: Viking, 1974.

U.S. Department of Health, Education and Welfare. *FDA Consumer.* H.E.W. publication no. (FDA) 79–2108, (July–August, 1978).

Valnet, Jean. *Heal Yourself with Vegetables, Fruits and Grains.* New York: Simon and Schuster, 1975.

Verrett, Jacqueline, and **Carper, J.** *Eating May Be Hazardous to Your Health.* New York: Simon and Schuster, 1974.

Wigmore, Ann. *Be Your Own Doctor.* Boston: Hippocrates Health Institute, 1972.

——. *Why Suffer?* Boston: Hippocrates Health Institute, 1964.

Williams, Roger J. *Nutrition against Disease: Environmental Prevention.* New York: Bantam, 1971.

Winter, Ruth. *A Consumer's Dictionary of Food Additives.* New York: Crown Press, 1978.

Yudkin, John, M.D. *Sweet and Dangerous.* New York: Bantam, 1972.

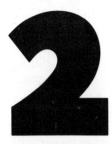

ALTERNATIVE
BIRTHING

Definition

We have included natural childbirth in this book because it is revolutionizing the process of birthing in the United States and is influencing changes in obstetrics and birth philosophy around the world. Numerous new delivery techniques have evolved that include the basic groundwork established by Lamaze. Concerned practitioners absorbed beliefs put forth by Lamaze to create additional natural birthing processes based upon safe, natural delivery, cooperation of parents and physicians, and feeling for the newborn.

The *Lamaze method* was developed by Dr. Fernand Lamaze after observing the procedure in Russia in 1951. He was so impressed by the conditioned-reflex method that Dr. Lamaze returned to France to teach, train, and use the method. *Montrices* (nurse educators) were trained to help the doctor and teach the method to parents. Needless to say, his method was considered quite radical by the French people, even though it was being used extensively in Europe and China. It was not until women had successfully delivered their babies and told others about it that the method was slowly accepted by Dr. Lamaze's colleagues.

But Dr. Lamaze was not the only one making use of natural childbirth or what is considered a modification of Pavlov's conditioning method. An English physician, Dr. Grantly Dick-Read, was also employing the theory of conditioning in childbirth. *Dick-Read's method is* similar to the Lamaze method. Both men felt that education about the body and its processes would help women understand childbirth, and conditioning exercises would aid relaxation and preparation during labor. Incorporating breathing exercises and practice, women could consciously deliver their babies without the use of debilitating drugs.

These two philosophies gained popularity in the fifties, and by 1959, the American Society of Psychoprophylaxis in Obstetrics, Inc., was established. Now there are many modifications and extensions of the Pavlov theory based on the procedures of these two pioneers in natural childbirth. A number of doctors have developed their own method of natural birthing and will train interested parents in his or her method of delivery. Furthermore, many holistically oriented centers have grown out of natural birthing and stress the interrelationship between spirit, mind, and body of parents and child.

All natural birthing methods educate both the father and the mother. Parents are taught to recognize and understand the pregnant body and its processes. Obstetricians denote that much of this education may be reeducation to "clean out" any misconceptions held by mother and father. The mother is taught exercises to tone up her body and prepare it for the birth process. The father coordinates these exercises by being a coach, a timer, and an acute observer. The goals of natural birthing are the same: to teach what to expect and how to prepare so that parents can approach their special event with calmness, actively participate with confidence, and take pride in the fact that they deliver a healthy baby with minor aid from hospital personnel.

The doctor, nurse, and father are supporters of the mother, as are family members and friends. Educational classes provide parents with experience and practice of the method and knowledge of the actual process. A mother controls delivery and experiences dignity in labor. The father is vital to the birth; he is naturally brought closer to the process and sees his wife with a deeper appreciation. This has rarely been acknowledged in the past.

Although many mothers declare that giving birth naturally was *less* painful than a hospital delivery, alternative birthing methods do not teach mothers that childbirth is painless. Many consumers are fearful of the discomfort involved in delivery and have erected long-standing barriers against the agony. For this reason a major focus of childbirth education is centered around pain. Parents are taught that their conceptions of discomfort during childbirth may be based upon stories told by others, experiences retold by others, uncertainty about what to expect, or fear of labor pains. Each of these ideas is treated as valid, but instructors seek to remove them by presenting facts that emphasize how individuals can control severe discomfort. Through varying techniques expectant mothers are informed about methods to refocus the mind away from the ordeal of labor.

Another commonality among natural birthing methods is education about drugs. Obstetricians point out that many of today's parents are concerned about the range of effects of drugs on the unborn and newly born child. Most natural delivery practitioners prefer that expecting mothers refrain from reliance upon drugs during delivery. Researchers report that "Valium administered to mothers during labor can still be found in the tissues of their newborn infants ten days after birth." (Haire, 1978). Thus drugs may hamper a newborn infant's resistance to diseases that confront him or her in the "new world" into which he or she is born. However, educators stress that drugs can always be used if pain is unbearable.

Medications taken after birth may not only affect the milk of a mother who is nursing but may also affect the child. If a mother decides to take anesthesia during delivery, she may be combining the problems. Dr. Yvonne Brackbill of the Georgetown University School of Medicine warns: "After the baby is born and must depend on its own bodily functions to detoxify drugs remaining in its system after birth, the rapidly developing nervous system is even more vulnerable to environmental insults (drugs, forceps, spinal taps, puncturing of fluids) which will re-route or alter the neurological development of the child" (Haire, 1978).* And, as pointed out by the Committee on Drugs of the American Academy of Pediatrics, "There is no drug, whether prescription or over-the-counter remedy, that has been proven safe for the unborn child."

Natural birthing methods meàn hard work. Parents must practice deligently outside class to perfect exercises and breathing techniques in order to consummate the birth procedure, so it is not easy. Practice time will have to be regimented to enable mother and partner to feel that the method becomes a natural procedure. Parents must master drills devoted to relaxing, exercising, breathing, visualization and meditation, and communication. Practice sessions are critical in making responses into reflexes. Timing, speed, accuracy, communication, and a feel for the body and newborn are employed simultaneously and must be well understood by birthing partners.

Information regarding alternative birthing is usually obtained in the pamphlets given to expectant mothers by an attending physician. However, do not be surprised if a physician does not recommend natural delivery. If this is a problem and a mother prefers natural childbirth, physicians can suggest someone who does encourage it. Many physicians are hesitant to deliver new babies without the aid of anesthesiologists and with help from parents. Still other practitioners will urge parents to attend specified classes purely for the physical and educational benefits.

Breakthroughs in natural childbirth have expanded personal and scientific understanding of these processes in ways that are only alluded to with a summary of natural birthing methods. Partners and practitioners alike have included much broader meanings to such words as *parenting, conscious control, feelings of the unborn,* and *communication.* Experience with the intricate inner workings of mother and child has spurred beliefs in the interrelationship of the spirit, mind, and body. Symbols of this are seen in educational classes within public health settings provided by hospitals and other associations. Further, pain research with biofeedback and acupuncture supports the birthing principle teaching: that the brain can control pain. A thesaurus of information from varying fields promotes communication links heretofore unexpected.

Since we began this chapter with the emergence of natural childbirth (Lamaze and Dick-Read) and the discussion of the traits prevalent in many alternative birthing practices, we felt it would be helpful to explain some of the lesser-known birth methods so that consumers become aware of the wide range of choices available. The differences between the methods are minor. All natural birthing practices seek to increase the meaningfulness of birth and cooperative, informed participation between parents and health care professionals.

Natural birthing approaches are also known as prepared childbirth. Frederich LeBoyer, a French physician, added another dimension to prepared birthing. The *LeBoyer method* of natural childbirth is quite different from others because it emphasizes the baby's transition from the womb to life. He reasoned that birth, when carried out in bright lights, with loud noises and jerky routines, frightened the newborn infant. To LeBoyer, the newborn's cries were indicative of the fear he or she experienced during birth and in a new environment.

The LeBoyer method welcomes the newborn. The baby is gradually introduced into his or her new environment by continuing the sensations the baby feels while in the uterus. Mother and partner develop expertise in breath coordination during education classes. They also receive instruction about parenting, nutrition, and physical, emotional, and spiritual interactions between parent and child.

Light and sound are major focuses of LeBoyer. During delivery, lights are kept dim so that the newborn's eyes are protected. Delivery room communication between parents and practitioner is smooth and consistent, requiring little sound. Baby hears muffled noises while in the uterus. Delivery in silence or with only the sound of whispers assures the newborn that passage into another existence is not threatening.

Partners are encouraged to deliver their child slowly for a number of reasons. Although some labor periods last longer than others, teachers of the LeBoyer method explain that the mother does not often tear herself from "pushing." They also assert that the placenta is expelled with greater ease because the body is consciously involved and aware when birth is complete. For baby, breathing is a new addition to his or her processes. Slow delivery allows the newborn to adapt to breathing in a more natural manner. The baby is placed on the mother's abdomen while breathing through both the umbilical cord and the nose. During this time, the baby is handled delicately; he or she is not inverted, swatted on the bottom, and rushed to the nursery. According to LeBoyer, the life energy flows through the spine. Routine birthing practices encountered by the newborn in hospitals can obstruct his or her life energy. Slow breathing and delivery methods coupled with emphasis on "special" treatment of the spine are two other focuses in LeBoyer.

Touch is still another accent of the LeBoyer method of natural childbirth. The baby's prebirth environment is slippery and soft. Upon delivery the naked newborn is placed on mother's abdomen and thus is reassured that the new environment is friendly, warm, and loving. Mother and father place a hand on the newborn's back to relay through touch the love and closeness felt for baby. The baby is turned on each side until he or she is comfortable in these positions before the mother props the baby up. The LeBoyer philosophy teaches that the baby's feelings are most important during the first few minutes of life.

The baby's next transitional experience is a warm bath. The newborn is slowly emerged up to the neck. Once again, he or she is in an environment similar to the uterus. Because of the body's buoyancy, the baby's arms and legs move freely. The bath lasts from three to six minutes, and then the baby is returned to mother. Practitioners affirm LeBoyer's belief that the newborn, if not already relaxed by the previous practices, immediately becomes calm when placed in the bath.

LeBoyer teaches that the baby has lived in a moving environment for nine months and is frightened by the stillness he or she feels after birth. Thus, parents are urged to walk or rock the baby often in order to soothe their baby's panic. As we have described, the baby is introduced to new situations gradually, receiving continual support and encouragement from parents.

Nurse-midwifery is another option available to expecting parents who wish to deliver their child by natural means. Nurse-midwives are available for home, hospital, or family center birth and provide parents with both preparation and specialized service. The nurse-midwife works with the family throughout the term of pregnancy. Even though these specialists must receive post-graduate training, there are many hospitals that will not allow nurse-midwives to deliver the newborn. For this reason you have to locate a practitioner through Family Centered Maternity Care or through local independent nurse practitioner agencies.

Mothers who have delivered with the help of a nurse-midwife state that they were asked if they had any questions *before* being given an examination or extra information. After answering questions, disseminating information, and examining the mother, a midwife explains that she has specialists on call for emergencies and months to prepare the whole family for birth. Since the nurse-midwife is trained to perform gynecological exams, mothers do not have to visit physicians unless they wish to be double-checked.

Nurse-midwives provide discussion and education about a varied number of topics that may be of interest to parents. These topics are arranged under a loose agenda, allowing parents to choose subjects for instruction. Nurse-midwives prepare both parents for the birth process with breathing techniques and pelvic exercises. They explain that in normal childbirth the body "knows" what to do. Parents must learn to follow the natural or instinctive inclinations of the body in addition to trusting its ability. The mother is asked to make contact with the baby through focused concentration and/or meditation. Parents learn a large body of information about self-care practices, infant care, body changes, nutrition, and future plans for birth control.

One of the attributes of the nurse-midwife is that he or she joins the parents early in the labor process rather than during the last stage, as is the general practice of the other prepared birthing methods. One mother, who had delivered her first child by the Lamaze method and her second child by the LeBoyer method, delivered her third child with the aid of a nurse-midwife at home. When we asked her to compare her three experiences, she stated that she preferred the nurse-midwife approach. She related that she felt that she and her husband had received more personal attention and had been treated more like "human beings instead of babymakers." In addition, she pointed out, the nurse-midwife was "mother conscious," which sharply differed from their previous "baby conscious" experiences.

Family Centered Maternity Care (FCMC) is a combination of professional care, prepared delivery, and shared family experience. Furthermore, family maternity centers seek to bring the comfort of home into the delivery and postdelivery setting. Their service is individualized in that parents are able to state their wishes ahead of time and the center will attempt to fulfill their birthing desires.

Birthing centers offer the equipment, a professional staff (doctors and nurses) for comfort, emergency situations, and consultation, and a family atmosphere designed by expecting parents. Parent education programs prepare fathers as partners, assistants, and coaches before, during, and after birth. Mothers learn breathing and toning exercises. Classes are available in nutrition, prenatal and postnatal care, and a variety of birth preparation methods and services through advocate organizations (La Leche League and International Childbirth Education Associations). In most cases, Family Centered Maternity Care is incorporated within the hospital itself.

The birthing process is a shared family experience. The father is not only permitted in the labor room, he is also given the opportunity to be at the mother's side during delivery; this directly contrasts with Lamaze, Dick-Read, and LeBoyer methods of natural childbirth *within the hospital setting*. Since fathers are often granted unlimited visiting privileges after birth, he shares the responsibility of caring for the newborn. The newborn is not separated from the mother after birth (unless she requests it or feels the need). This allows the baby to room in with mother. The father and, in some FCMC units, older children are also allowed to room in with the mother after birth.

Delivering your child at home is the final birth alternative we will discuss. Home delivery can be accomplished by the mother and father with the support of friends or a qualified professional. However, Lamaze and Dick-Read teachers and physicians do not recommend home birth, whereas LeBoyer assistants and nurse-midwives will deliver in the home environment. The major drawback for parents wishing to deliver their baby at home is that many obstetricians do not support home birth. Natural birth at home is considered by its proponents to be the traditional and most comfortable environment for parents and newborn. Advocates of home birth point out that regardless of the natural delivery technique employed (Lamaze, LeBoyer, Dick-Read, or other preparations), home delivery is a safe and natural act.

Whether you attend a prepared birthing course or individualized instruction for home birth, parents train together. In home delivery the spiritual nature of birth is emphasized. Coaching, breathing, toning, sanitizing, gathering of necessary equipment, relaxing, birthing processes, nutrition, meditation, and body coordination are some examples of educational instructions parents receive for home delivery. As with the other alternative delivery methods, classes are intensive and last for at least six weeks.

There are two interesting points regarding the last stages of labor, which are brought out during the instruction in home birth. One of these is that the mother should walk around while having labor pains. According to one mother, walking shortened her labor time. She was told that the pull of gravity would hasten the baby's delivery. Another mother told us that a warm bath eased her pain and body weight. She was instructed to do breathing exercises until she dialated to eight centimeters. She followed her teacher's recommendations, hopped out of the tub, and delivered her baby with great ease. This mother further asserted that a bath can prevent mother from having to be cut before delivery because the skin is more flexible and easily stretched. Being prepared to deliver a child at home by natural means is the most recent movement in alternative birthing procedures. Parents who have experienced home birth promise that it is "the only way to go."

The following table lists the characteristics of each of these techniques for natural birth. We suggest that the consumer examine this information in order to decide upon a particular preference and then pursue your choice by reading the relevant books listed at the end of the chapter. Instructors for each of the methods we have discussed should be certified in his or her particular birthing method. This means that they have taken instruction from the parent organization and have passed an examination, as in the case of Lamaze, or they have received formal training and certification, as in the case of nurse-midwifery. All methods propose to educate parents, although some do not provide instruction regarding parenting skills, nutrition, and postnatal care, among other areas. As you shall learn in the next section, alternative birthing methods can be purely "natural" or natural with built-in options for qualified medical professionals and treatment.

Type of Healing

Not all the alternatives available to parents are completely natural. In fact even though the mother and father are prepared actually to deliver the baby by natural means, the father is often excluded from the delivery and assumes a subordinate role. Parents choosing Lamaze, Dick-Read, and nurse-midwifery are usually told that anesthesia is available during the last moments of delivery for mothers in pain. Additionally, it is recommended that natural means be used *only* for "normal" deliveries and that obstetricians are required for the delivery. Nurse-midwives, however, will deliver without the aid of a physician, and the choice of being anesthesized is left to the mother.

Family Centered Maternity Care units are also crossovers. Because these maternity centers are usually located within the hospital, a distinction between natural delivery and scientific medical care appears vague. Additionally, services are available to parents after birth. Should

Characteristics of Alternative Birthing Methods

Birthing Method	Breathing Techniques	Exercise and Body Toning	Self-Care Practices	Partner Co-Operation	Parenting	Nutrition	Sanitation	Meditation	Pre-Natal Care	Post-Natal Care	Spiritual Emphasis	Touch	Family Oriented	Gradual Delivery	Walk During Labor	Bath During Labor	Built-in Safety	Used Only In Hospital	Applicable To Home Or Hospital
Lamaze	X	X		X					X								X	X[b]	
Dick-Read	X	X		X	X				X								X	X[b]	
LeBoyer	X	X		X		X	X		X	X	X	X	X	X			X		X
Nurse-Midwife	X	X	X	X	X	X	X	X	X	X			X	X[a]	X	X	X		X
Home Birth	X	X	X	X	X	X	X		X	X	X	X	X	X			X		X
FCMC	X	X	X	X	X	X			X	X			X				X	X	

[a]Some nurse-midwives encourage gradual delivery and some do not.

[b]These methods have been employed at home without the consent of physicians.

parents desire a totally natural experience for their birth event, this alternative will not suit that requirement.

LeBoyer and home birth (along with some nurse-midwife services) offer partners a satisfying, natural birthing alternative. LeBoyer instructors deliver babies at home upon request (but check with your attending physician), bring the equipment needed for birth, and do not advocate the use of drugs. Home birth methods (which include LeBoyer techniques) encompass information, instruction about preparing the home environment, and aid for families during delivery. Parents supply the equipment for delivery and direct the process in their own environment. *Regardless of the birthing choice, all parents should alert an obstetrician when labor begins in case of emergency.*

The methods of a nurse-midwife combine all the other procedures. Anesthesia is available, but they prefer natural delivery; they will deliver without the assistance of a physician and will deliver in the home environment. Parents are not totally responsible for home delivery apparatus. However, the nurse-midwife does not care for the family after birth, as in Family Centered Maternity Care programs. (The other methods discussed also exclude care after pregnancy except through education of postnatal care.)

All of the birth alternatives include breathing techniques to focus the mind and coordinate with the body's processes. Prenatal care and partner cooperation are emphasized as much as exercise and body toning practices during preparation before birth. Although not specifically stated as such, these educational procedures imply that individual responsibility is an important component of natural childbirth. Built-in safety practices accompany all methods in that each procedure prepares parents for emergencies. Safety measures include a stand-in physician for complications, anesthesia in case of discomfort and proper sanitation and equipment, in addition to the prepared awareness of partners.

Description of Method

Expertise in alternative birthing practices is acquired through classes and achieved by the hard work of both parents. The first set of classes will educate parents about the body and what happens to it during pregnancy, childbirth, and the postnatal period, through diagrams, slides, pictures, lectures, and personal experiences. In addition, parents will learn about the labor process, muscle toning exercises, breathing exercises, pain and—in some methods—parenting, nutrition, and birth control. Prenatal and postnatal care are also discussed, but some methods, as mentioned earlier, are more complete in their education than others.

Parents usually attend six to twelve classes depending upon the approach. Teachers of prepared methods have specific points to address during each class, and one or both parents are required to attend every class. In nurse-midwifery parents (usually just the mother) choose the educational topics from a varied list and receive class instruction according to choice. FCMC services also expand the educational information to parents by providing continuous services before, during, and after pregnancy.

Perhaps one of the greatest contributions to childbirth was the correlation of breathing to contractions. Regardless of the birth method, breathing procedures are the mainstay of the program. Through breathing, the mother creates an alternative line of concentration during labor as well as communicates directly with the natural birth-giving processes of the body. In some methods relaxation and meditation are used in conjunction with breathing techniques. The mother achieves some control over herself, we are told, and therefore some control over the labor process and birth. Training begins by learning how to breathe correctly and naturally and moves into controlling breath for specific labor periods.

It is through breathing methods that parents realize the necessity for practice. Breath must be mastered, for it is not an easy feat to decide upon a stage of labor and automatically breathe the correct way. The mother must also remain relaxed during her labor process. The responsibility for breathing control, relaxing, and timing is shared with her partner, who should guide her through labor. Instructors of most alternative birthing practices acknowledge that parents are encouraged to practice once a day to perfect exercises for toning and breathing. Practicing exercises takes a great deal of time, but once they are mastered by partners, time can be cut in half.

The father or partner is intimately involved in both exercise and breathing processes during practice sessions and the actual labor event. The birthing partner must accurately judge how relaxed the mother is, which exercise to use, when the mother should change breathing techniques, and which stage of labor she is in, and he must decide when to go to the hospital or ready the home delivery area. All methods stress that the partner provide the majority of moral and physical support. He must be as prepared as the mother, which involves his understanding bodily processes and pregnancy stages. During labor he relays the commands for breathing as well as reports the progress on the delivery to the mother. In home birth classes he must also be able to deliver the newborn. The father is not only a sounding board and a director for the mother, he also acts as an intermediary between the physician (and attending personnel) and mother in the labor and delivery rooms. But in LeBoyer and home birth, the father is truly an equal partner in delivery.

Instructors of Lamaze, Dick-Read, and home birthing methods

suggest that parents practice with the attending physician or practitioner and partner *before* labor. In this way, they point out, all participants of the delivery simulate the labor process, increase efficiency, and establish direct lines of communication. However, many times physicians are unable to do this. According to instructors, if this happens to be the case with the attending obstetrician, a mother will find her partner to be the greatest help during delivery. Since he will be able to watch exactly what is happening and has practiced before the delivery, the partner will be able to guide the mother through the birth.

Fear of pain is handled by educating parents about the causes of pain, providing exercises to decrease pain by toning up the body, teaching techniques to change the focus of concentration during pain and breathing techniques to promote relaxation and body ease. Through these, a mother becomes self-confident while approaching labor so that she is no longer tense or afraid. Many parents tell us that their only control over the birth process before natural birthing methods was at the time of the actual conception. Prepared childbirth classes teach that parents are in control of the whole birthing process and that it is their right to question the physician or hospital facilities.

For parents and consumers it is important to ask questions, explore the alternatives, and decide which is best for both parents and newborn child. Many physicians have their own method of natural birthing they wish to use. But before you choose an alternative birthing method, we suggest you read over the questions in the following box so that they can be answered during your research.

Questions for Parents Seeking Alternative Birthing Methods

1. How much total care do we want as parents?
2. How will the doctor or practitioner comply with our wishes?
3. How much time will be spent away from our newborn?
4. How much time will be spent away from the family?
5. Where do we want to deliver our newborn?
6. What type of instructional courses or sessions are available to partners?
7. What facilities are available for emergencies?
8. How many classes must be attended and at what time?
9. What kinds of medicines may be involved?
10. How much control are we given during delivery?
11. Can all of our personal needs be met by the method?
12. Does the cost of instruction include delivery?

It is crucial to consider every possibility when bringing another person into the world. To bring a baby into the world safely and happily should be the ultimate goal. There are many other related facilities available to parents, as well as a number of qualified professionals ready to educate them. All natural birthing methods assert that having a baby is extremely individualized; no two persons have a baby in exactly the same way. For this reason, it is best for consumers to remember that birthing classes teach what happens to the "average" person; there is no "going by the book" when having a baby.

Duration of Treatment

As we have mentioned earlier, classes in prepared methods will last six weeks, although a few methods vary somewhat. The class period is usually two hours in length once a week for six consecutive weeks. Practice sessions between partners are scheduled at home and generally require one hour each night at first, but they are recommended for the entire carrying period.

If parents have not yet decided to have a child by natural means, they may be encouraged to know that it is possible to begin instruction for prepared methods at any time during pregnancy, even though LeBoyer and home birth methods prefer that partners begin early. It will be easier, according to mothers, to practice exercises in the first months, but this does not mean that it is impossible to practice after that time. In fact, some prepared classes are so overbooked that they have to start many mothers as late as seven and a half months. In any event, teachers point out, body tone, enhanced through birthing practices, relieves some of the stress associated with carrying extra body weight and provides for natural weight loss after pregnancy. One mother who began instruction in Lamaze right before her eighth month felt that the exercise and breathing techniques gave her great relief during her final month. She said, "They cleared my mind every day and made my body feel like I had done something." By the way, she succeeded in having a healthy baby by natural means.

Most of the Lamaze and Dick-Read classes provide only education and body-centered instructions. LeBoyer, nurse-midwifery, home birth preparations, and Family Centered Maternity Care include both nutritional education and parenting. Even though teachers of Lamaze and Dick-Read preparations state that they are primarily focusing upon relaxation and conditioned reflexes before and during labor, we feel that the exclusion of parenting and nutrition education within their frameworks leaves a job only half done.

Cost Range

    Lamaze—$25–$40
    Dick-Read—$25–$35
    LeBoyer—$50–$250 (for home delivery)
    Nurse-midwife—$250–$350 (for home delivery)
    Home birth—$200–$250
    Family Centered Maternity Care—$500–$1,000

Personal Responsibilities

Personal responsibilities regarding prepared methods are numerous. First, parents are expected to attend every meeting of scheduled classes. If parents already have children, arrangements will have to be made so that participation in class is possible. A flexible baby-sitter would be to your advantage in case class runs late. Second, times are not always variable. For instance, they may be scheduled only at night. Unless job hours coincide, it will be difficult for parents working a night shift to attend. Some parents, therefore, may have to make temporary changes in work schedules.

Primarily it is the parents' duty to practice. This is the biggest responsibility to all prepared methods and to the unborn child. Parents are encouraged to practice at least once a day and will have to schedule practice sessions for at least an hour's time. Most parents find this the hardest requirement to fulfill. Parents with children try to wait until they are in bed and then find themselves too tired to practice. Partners may find it easier to practice an hour before supper while also teaching the children.

Parents are also responsible for choosing the attending practitioner and practicing the procedure with him or her before actually giving birth. Many physicians who have referred expectant parents to prepared birthing classes are aware of what is expected. But if an obstetrician cannot fulfill this suggestion, it is the partners' responsibility to make sure the doctor knows the communication system established by you. Along these lines, some LeBoyer physicians are hesitant about home birth. Should you prefer birth at home with the LeBoyer method, prepare to ask your practitioner if he or she objects to this instead of making assumptions. Note, too, that obstetricians are trained to spot problems and subvert emergencies. Fathers, then, should not attempt to overtake that role. Many hospitals do not allow fathers in the delivery room, nor do they have rooms prepared for natural childbirth, even though physicians are allowed to deliver by natural means. The family structure, an integral component of birth, may have to be sacrificed due to lack of space or available rooms. Although this may be disheartening, there are alternatives—in birthing centers, clinics, and private practices. If you decide upon natural childbirth during early pregnancy, you have a great deal of time to investigate these aspects and to choose other possibilities. If hospital facilities do not meet your needs, the organizations listed in this chapter can help you find what you require for maternity services.

Practitioners promoting natural birthing measures often require parents to sign an informed-consent form before prepared birth instruction begins. This form states the responsibilities of both parties (partners and physician), in addition to possible dangers. Practitioners point out that the form is not legally binding, but because natural childbirth is still considered a "new" procedure, it is beneficial in establishing communication lines.

As we discussed earlier, teachers of these alternative birthing methods must be certified. Ask your potential instructor where he or she received training and how long he or she has been teaching and/or practicing the method. If the instructor does not have any proof of qualifications, find another. It will also be beneficial to discuss with your partner what you want from an alternative method. Reread the questions we presented earlier so that a method agreeable to both of you is chosen.

It is especially important for unmarried mothers to choose a partner who will accept the responsibilities of practice, class attendance, and cooperation during pregnancy. Partners are equally involved in natural birthing methods, which require hard work, support, concern, communication, and caring.

Home birthing practices place more responsibility upon consumers than the other methods we discuss. Partners must alter the environment, procure necessary equipment and sanitized utensils, and be consciously aware of the body and its processes during pregnancy. As a safety precaution, be certain to contact a professional as soon as labor *begins* so that he or she is prepared for emergencies. Call after the baby is born and let him or her know that the delivery was a success.

Finally, the responsibility for baby's health is very important. Even though nutrition is not directly stressed in some birthing classes, it is crucial that parents learn something about the relationship between good nutrition and a healthy baby. We urge parents to research the subject and implement the practices of scientific nutrition during and after pregnancy.

Informational Organizations

American Society for Psychoprophylaxis in Obstetrics, Inc.
1523 L Street, NW, Suite 104
Washington, DC 20005

LaLeche League International
9616 Minneapolis Avenue
Franklin Park, IL 60131

American College of Home Obstetrics
664 N. Michigan Avenue, Suite 610
Chicago, IL 60611

American College of Nurse-Midwives
1000 Vermont Avenue, NW
Washington, DC 20005

National Association of Parents and Professionals
for Safe Alternatives in Childbirth
PO Box 1307
Chapel Hill, NC 27514

Consistencies

1. Practitioners and instructors attempt to avoid relying upon anesthesia by teaching self-reliance through natural techniques. This philosophy is thereby consistent with a major tenet of holism: personal responsibility. The patient or consumer is no longer totally dependent upon the physician. Rather, they establish an interdependence and cooperation in the birthing process.

2. Classes in natural birthing teach partners about the techniques used for the process. Fathers play an important role as members of the delivery team. This leads to shared experiences and is meaningful for both parents rather than just being the sole province of the mother. The long-term effects of this practice would seem to increase the interest of the male partner in the child. Most families feel a deep spiritual commitment to each other and to the child after a "natural" birth.

3. Alternatives can reduce medical costs because anesthesiologists and other supporting personnel do not have to be present during delivery. Since the average cost of having a baby can range between $1,500 and $2,500, with the anesthesiologist charging between $250 and $500, prepared birth can make a big difference in the total amount of the bill.

4. Breakthroughs in natural childbirth brought about by Lamaze have expanded scientific understanding of the "natural" delivery process and, as an indirect consequence, holistic health. That pain can be consciously controlled indicates that it is possible to gain control of bodily processes, which can facilitate many other health measures.

5. A large number of obstetricians who make use of prepared birth advocate the informed-consent form so that consumers are aware of assets and deficiencies of the method as well as responsibilities.

Inconsistencies

1. Some birthing methods omit the basic principles of nutrition and its importance for prenatal and postnatal care. This is inconsistent with the holistic perspective and represents a narrow approach to health maintenance. Holistic physicians object to this neglect of the total life situation of the individual.

2. There are no long-range studies correlating these methods with the degree of pain experienced by mothers. It is surprising that, with all the literature available on alternative birthing methods, a study of this kind has not been conducted.

3. Though natural delivery is an important step in having a baby, it is unfortunate that many methods do not incorporate continuing instruction after the birth is complete. Once again, this implies that they miss an important opportunity to implement holistic methods as a continuation of the educational process of health maintenance.

4. Some birthing classes are only scheduled at night. Consequently, those who work at night are automatically excluded from the education-experiential process. Instructors need to develop more flexible schedules so that those who work at night can participate.

Sources to Read

Arms, Suzanne. *Immaculate Deception: A New Look at Women and Childbirth in America.* Boston: Houghton Mifflin, 1975.

Bauman, Edward, et al. *The Holistic Health Handbook.* Berkeley, CA: And/Or Book Press, 1978.

Bing, Elisabeth. *Experiences in the Lamaze Method of Prepared Childbirth.* New York: Ace Books, 1970.

———. *Six Practical Lessons for an Easier Childbirth.* New York: Bantam, 1967.

Bonstein, Isadore, M.D. *Psychoprophylactic Preparation for Painless Childbirth.* London: William Heinemann Medical Books, 1958; and New York: Grune and Stratton, 1958.

Boston Woman's Health Book Collective. *Our Bodies, Ourselves.* New York: Simon and Schuster, 1976.

Bradley, Robert A. *Husband-Coached Childbirth.* New York: Harper and Row, 1974.

Brewer, Gail and **Tom.** *What Every Pregnant Woman Should Know about Diet and Drugs in Pregnancy.* New York: Random House, 1977.

Bricklin, Alice G. *Mother Love: The Book of Natural Child Rearing.* Philadelphia: Running Press, 1975.

Brook, Danae. *Naturebirth: You, Your Body, and Your Baby.* New York: Pantheon, 1976.

Chabon, Irwin, M.D. *Awake and Aware: Participating in Childbirth through Psychoprophylaxis.* New York: Dell, 1979.

Dick-Read, Grantley. *Childbirth without Fear.* New York: Harper and Row, 1944.

Eiger, Marvio, and **Olds, Karen.** *The Complete Book of Breastfeeding.* New York: Workman, 1972.

Eloesser, Leo; Galt, Edity J.; and **Hemingway, Isabel.** *Pregnancy, Childbirth, and the Newborn: A Manual for Rural Midwives.* Mexico City: Instituto Indigesta Inter-Americano, 1959.

Ewy, Donna and Roger. *Preparation for Childbirth: A Lamaze Guide.* Boulder, CO: Pruett, 1970.

Gaskin, Ina May. *Spiritual Midwifery.* Summertown, TN: Book Publishing Co., 1977.

Goodrich, Frederick, Jr., M.D. *Natural Childbirth.* Englewood Cliffs, NJ: Prentice-Hall, 1956.

Haire, Doris B. "A New Look at Drug Abuse in Childbirth," in *Wholistic Dimensions in Healing: A Resource Guide.* by Leslie J. Kaslof. New York: Doubleday and Company, Inc., 1978.

Hazell, Lester Dessez. *Commonsense Childbirth.* New York: Berkeley, 1976.

Kaslof, Leslie J. *Wholistic Dimensions in Healing.* Garden City, NY: Doubleday, 1978.

Kitzinger, Shelia. *The Experience of Childbirth.* New York: Taplinger, 1972.

Lamaze, Fernand. *Painless Childbirth,* trans. Denise Lloyd. New York: Pocket Books, 1972.

Lang, Raven. *Birth Book.* Ben Lomond, CA: Genesis Press, 1972.

Leboyer, Frederick. *Birth without Violence.* New York: Alfred A. Knopf, 1975.

Marzolla, Jean, ed. *9 Months 1 Day 1 Year.* New York: Harper and Row, 1975.

Myers, Margaret F. *A Textbook for Midwives.* London: Churchill Livingstone, 1972.

Newton, Niles. *The Family Book of Child Care.* New York: Harper and Row, 1957.

Nilsson, Ingleman-Sundberg and Wirsen. *A Child Is Born.* New York: Dell, 1969.

Noble, Elizabeth. *Essential Exercises for the Childbearing Year.* Boston: Houghton Mifflin, 1976.

Raphel, Dana. *The Tender Gift: Breastfeeding.* Englewood Cliffs, NJ: Prentice-Hall, 1973.

Rich, Adrienne. *Of Woman Born: Motherhood As Experience and Institution.* New York: Norton, 1976.

Shaw, Nancy Stoller. *Forced Labor: Maternity Care in the United States.* Elmsford, NY: Pergamon Press, 1974.

Sousa, Marion. *Childbirth at Home.* Englewood Cliffs, NJ: Prentice-Hall, 1976.

Stewart, David and Lee, eds. *Safe Alternatives in Childbirth.* Chapel Hill, NC: National Association of Parents and Professionals for Safe Alternatives in Childbirth, 1978.

Tanzer, Deborah. *Why Natural Childbirth?* New York: Doubleday, 1972.

Vellay, Pierre, M.D. *Childbirth with Confidence.* New York: Macmillan, 1969.

Ward, Charlotte and Fred. *The Home Birth Book.* Washington, DC: INSCAPE Publishers, 1976.

Wesses, Helen. *Natural Childbirth and the Family.* New York: Harper and Row, 1973.

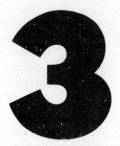

NATUROPATHY

Definition

Naturopathy became a distinct healing practice during the early part of this century. Dr. Benjamin Lust founded this new field of healing when he met with practitioners of *hydrotherapy*, and the group decided to expand the water cure to include *all natural* methods of treating disease used at the time. Such measures as homoeopathy, herbalism, manipulation, nutrition, psychology, and medical electricity were incorporated along with hydrotherapy into the field of naturopathy. These practitioners, who became known as naturopaths, believed that dis-ease was caused by violations of natural laws.

Naturopathy "is medicine for people, not for diseases" (National College of Naturopathic Medicine, 1981–82; Hewlett-Parsons, 1968; Tribe, 1968). This means that dis-ease is cured by examination and treatment of spiritual, mental, and physical components of the individual. These physicians note that imbalance in any one of these three major areas creates an imbalance in others. Dis-ease is seen as the manifestation of a number of problems and cannot be treated by mere removal of symptoms. Naturopathic practitioners search for the underlying causes of illness so that healing is accomplished on all levels of a person's life.

These holistic assumptions are based upon the natural law of homeostasis, a balanced state of spirit, mind, and body, which enables a person to adapt to change. In other words, the body contains the inherent ability to heal itself by way of the *vital force*. Practitioners emphasize natural means of reacting to stress harmonically through the innate forces of the body. They seek to prevent the occurrence of symptoms by attaining a dynamic balance of the entire person.

The vital force has vibrational qualities that create a balanced flux in the body. Abnormal vibrations on either physical, mental, or spiritual planes create a symptom that cannot adjust to change. The essential links to the vital force are earth (food), air, water, fire, and sound. These natural elements are the primary means employed to stimulate the natural process of homeostasis. Even though a wide variety of options are available for the treatment of dis-ease or imbalance, patients are believed to be unique and the practitioner must discover those methods related to the needs of each client.

Naturopaths are expected to develop expertise in both the scientific and natural modes of diagnosis and treatment. Thus, this field has both scientific validation and philosophically relevant foundations for a variety of healing modalities. Naturopaths are required to master the history, evidence, and current research available in each field and to integrate all of them into one system of healing. The students are trained as general practitioners and only rarely become specialists in any one healing modality. Minor surgical procedures are also a part of naturopathy, whereas major surgery is referred to surgical specialists. In addition to studying hydrotherapy, nutrition therapy, acupuncture, herbalism, homoeopathy, massage, and color therapy, naturopaths must also learn how to individualize these treatments to each consumer.

These healers, however, do not adhere to the doctrine that germs cause dis-ease. Instead, naturopaths emphasize that dis-ease leads to germs. Practitioners feel that consumers receive the benefits of a *complete* system of healing, which promotes health for each individual. The goal of this treatment is to cleanse and rebuild the client, in addition to teaching him or her to live in harmony with the self and the social and natural environment. In this way, naturopathy becomes a way of life for the consumer. Naturopaths teach these principles to the consumer in hopes of laying a foundation upon which health can be rebuilt. The healee joins the healer in designing and implementing a program to reshape the beliefs, actions, and habits of the client in order to promote health and maintain homeostasis.

Since healers in this field involve the client in every aspect of treatment, it is not easy for the consumer. Both time and money are involved, but, according to practitioners, optimum health is the benefit. A naturopath can remove the immediate symptoms, but he or she is primarily concerned with the "whys" underlying symptoms. These practitioners assert that a healee must actively work up to health with the motivation and confidence needed to generate change in daily routines. Bill Tribe (1978), noted naturopathic physician, affirms that naturopathic practitioners provide the client with "the means to achieve the highest possible level of health and encouragement to use them." Clients, then, are given the responsibility for attaining and maintaining well-being on a daily basis.

Currently, the legal restrictions placed on naturopathy are limiting consumers wishing to make use of this system of healing. There are only four states that allow licensed doctors to practice, twenty other states define specific boundaries in which naturopathy is practiced, and a few other states limit practice under common law. However, many states are changing these laws. Some practitioners record chiropractic as their specialty and include naturopathic components within their practice. We should point out that most states have naturopathic practitioners available for treatment of dis-ease. Following is a list of states that have granted naturopathic physicians practicing rights: Arizona, Connecticut, District of Columbia, Florida, Hawaii, Idaho, Kansas, North Carolina, Oregon, Utah, and Washington (Jennings, 1976).

Naturopathy is *not* just considered by its professionals as being an auxiliary therapy to other forms of treatment. Instead, it is a distinct method that makes use of both science and nature. However, healers join with orthodox physicians in cases that warrant it. It is precisely because of its multidimensionality that naturopathic physicians declare that they usually "cure" one who tries the method. The preventive nature of this method makes it one of the outstanding holistic practices, though there is little scientific support for these cures.

Prevention of disorders resides in those programs provided by practitioners and the natural measures adopted for home use. Patients are made aware of first aid methods in addition to hydrotherapy, massage, nutrition, exercise, and stress reduction techniques. Because many of these factors are employed as treatment, the patient can put them to use within an individualized plan for obtaining health. Naturopaths intend that the health program be included as regimen in order to maintain well-being. They point out that the ultimate power for the cure of disorders resides within the individual, not the practitioner. One may complete naturopathic treatment with restored health, but to remain free from dis-ease it is necessary for the patient to take active steps toward preserving well-being.

Just as we find in homoeopathy, practitioners rely upon the *law of cure model*. The law of cure states that symptoms leave the body in reverse order of appearance. That is, the most recent symptom leaves first, with the rest following in reverse chronological order. In order to be considered "cured," the symptoms that were present *before* the dis-ease was treated (or before it was serious enough to require a physician's treatment) must also reappear. The visibility of "old symptoms," termed *healing crisis* by naturopaths, means that the treatment is stimulating recuperative processes.

It is imperative that consumers understand the law of cure and healing crisis so that one does not believe that the disorder is serious. Let us say that you visit a naturopath and are diagnosed with a peptic ulcer. After initial treatment, pains in the stomach area disappear. Perhaps you experienced headaches, gastritis, nausea, and constipation before feeling stomach pain. Since each "healing crisis" is associated with each new set of symptoms, the crises in this example would be at the onset of constipation, followed by the onset of nausea, gastritis, and ending with headaches. After all symptoms related to the ulcer have been reexperienced, the disorder is termed "cured."

Under naturopathic treatment, our friend with the peptic ulcer would be requested to make a number of changes in his or her life so that future problems would be prevented. Practitioners suggest that each patient under care be prepared for intensive examination and rehabilitation in areas of vital concern. Naturopaths operate through treatment of the whole person. With the training, practice, and self-confidence instilled in the patient by this holistic practitioner, the integrated healing system of naturopathy can guide one to physical, mental, and spiritual well-being. Naturopathy is holistic in foundation and in character. It is the hope of naturopaths that their treatment enables one to experience the interrelationships of both internal and external factors as they are associated with health and disease.

Type of Healing

Since naturopathy is defined by the laws of nature and makes use of natural practices, it is considered a natural healing method by those within medicine. At the risk of sounding repetitious, we want to emphasize that the practice of naturopathy is holistic in both treatment and prevention. The use of natural remedies and techniques to stimulate the vital force promotes the body's own healing powers. Education and counseling also create consumer awareness of these processes.

Naturopathy, it is purported, is a multidimensional *system* of healing, which is practically impossible to divide into the categories outlined in this book. Type of method should point out to the reader why a healing method is natural or not. However, in naturopathy type of method will describe the types of natural methods employed in naturopathic treatment. Description of the method will explain not only the treatment process but also how these are applied to healing.

As mentioned before in the definition section of this chapter, naturopaths make use of much of the knowledge and practice of homoeopathy and herbalism. Medical preparations of substances may be employed to relieve symptoms, to stimulate the vital force, or to restore health. Furthermore, practitioners often suggest herbal teas as refreshment. They believe that natural medicaments do follow natural laws and thus are congruent with homeostasis. Healers point out that natural substances serve purposes other than stimulation of the vital force. They also promote elimination and assimilation of foods in addition to neutralizing toxins and wastes within the system, actions vital to homeostasis.

Naturopaths acquire more knowledge of scientific nutrition than physicians in standard medical schools because of nutrition's indispensable function in treatment and prevention of disorders. Practitioners affirm that the blood, providing necessary nutrients to all areas, is the life stream of the body and must furnish the correct balance and mixture of foods for well-being. Nutritional techniques are used to accomplish both cleansing and strengthening of the body. Healers do not believe that supplements should replace food. Although vitamins may be employed within treatment, it is preferred (by most physicians in the field) that food be used whenever possible to provide a balanced diet. The healee is encouraged to nourish the body with a variety of fresh vegetables, fresh fruits, dairy products, and meats. It is believed that all foods are needed in order to receive the proper balance of vitamins and minerals. These practitioners, therefore, do not advocate eliminating meats from the diet. But, consumer instruction in nutrition goes much further. The healee is also taught how to shop for fresh foods, how to cook and prepare foods, and how to eat and store them properly.

Many healers explain that quite often energy intake and dispersement have a bearing upon proper breathing. Patterns of breath affect the heart beat, which then influences the blood flow and its functions. Naturopaths employ deep breathing exercises and/or meditation in order to regulate rhythm. Furthermore, the healee is instructed on the relationships between breathing function and exercise, posture, mental state, and fresh air.

Within naturopathic medicine today, hydrotherapy still remains one of the primary tools for cleansing and nourishing the body. There are many methods within hydrotherapy available to the naturopath, some of which the consumer will most definitely experience. Douches, colonics, baths, fasting, packs, and/or compresses may be used for any dis-ease to stimulate the vital force. Elimination of toxins through bodily functions and expulsion of poisons through the skin, as well as dispersing inflammation and congestion, are the purposes of water therapy in naturopathy. According to practitioners, these techniques influence the body's self-heating mechanisms.

The prominence of exercise for establishing and maintaining vital energy is another natural area in naturopathic educational programs for the healee. Manipulation and massage techniques deliver the dual actions of driving blood to areas that need assistance and aid in expulsion of toxins. Naturopaths promote passive exercise through massage and manipulation programs that are designed according to individual eccentricities. Naturopaths declare that these types of treatments strengthen, restore, and preserve bodily capabilities in addition to correcting structural irregularities.

Many readers are probably aware that dry cell batteries have been employed by occult sciences for many years. Often combined with hydrotherapy and/or sound, the use of electricity as treatment in naturopathy stimulates metabolism. Healers are taught that underlying all life is a natural vibratory force made of electromagnetic energy. Electrical treatment initiates homeostasis through several methods. Naturopaths assert that the idea behind the battery is that galvanic (continuous) current stimulates metabolism and continues its action for several days after the treatment. Diathermy, a different form of electrical treatment, is a high-frequency current that produces heat in any part of the body and at any depth. Various other combinations are alternating currents of low voltage used in insulated hydrotherapeutic treatment, ultraviolet rays, and infrared and ultrasonic rays.

One of the most interesting natural measures employed in naturopathy is that of *chromotherapy*: the use of colors to heal. Practitioners point out that certain colors produce beneficial variations in a depleted system, perhaps because of their vibrational quality. However, color therapy is highly controversial at this time because some naturopaths feel that the colors are only conducive to psychological transformation rather than physiological change. Other practitioners point out that subsequent psychological change promotes concrete alterations on the physical realm. At this time, there is not enough conclusive research to settle these different opinions. For this reason, most naturopaths limit the use of chromotherapy as treatment. In the following list we have extracted some colors and their proposed actions as food for thought:

green—soothing to the nerves; as a visual symbol of life
red—stimulates nerves and blood
reddish-orange—inhibits malignant growths and aids in skin conditions
yellowish-orange—stimulates the digestive system
pillar box red—stimulates the male sex organs
navy blue—increases level of happiness
pastel blue—increases concentration and memory
orange—increases energy level; as a visual symbol of health

Self-awareness is an intimate aspect of naturopathic care. Self-concept, feelings, life-style characteristics, dreams, job satisfaction, and attitudes are a few of the personal segments used by holistic naturopaths to determine what contributes to the dis-eased state in each client. Education is blended into treatment for the purpose of producing and/or conserving the vital force. Practitioners affirm that health promotion must be more than a temporary vocation to adopt during dis-ease. Rather, they believe that health is an ongoing process that involves a patient's care and concern for spirit, mind, and body on a daily basis.

Naturopaths are of the belief that it is precisely because each individual is vitally different that naturopathy makes use of such a wide array of natural methods. Many techniques are embodied in an agenda designed to rouse the self-healing processes in the individual. The healthy individual as defined by practitioners in this field enjoys a balanced relationship with spiritual, mental, and physical facets of his or her life and thereby adapts to environment change with few problems of transition. Healers in naturopathy are sure that the science and art of medicine are synthesized in naturopathic healing. Natural essences of earth, air, water, fire, and sound intermix in order to provide consumers with what naturopaths believe to be the most multidimensional practice available in the field of health care.

Description of Healing Method

Now that we have presented you with the various natural methodologies naturopaths use, we must summarize how they are applied in this healing system. Homeostatic harmony is the vital force that holds the body's natural healing powers. Practitioners attempt to treat imbalances in such a manner that self-healing abilities are excited. Therefore, naturopaths explain that the patient cures him or herself and is only assisted by the naturopathic practitioner.

Naturopathic physicians pride themselves in performing extremely thorough examinations. A general physical will consist of the same types of tests given by any physician. Chemical testing is the second phase of examination, where healers examine the urine for an over-abundance or lack of nutrients in the body. Most practitioners point out that a urine test is not conclusive in itself; so consumers are often required to procure detailed hair and blood analysis in order to attain a complete chemical workup. Though the urine analysis is usually performed in a naturopath's office, other testing must be obtained elsewhere. The structural inspection of the spine is another exam required by naturopaths. A practitioner looks at the alignment of vertebrae for possible maladjustment and observes how one performs during walking, sitting, running, and standing for further information about posture.

The tests will not end, however, the quest for the underlying causes of disease. Healers in this field, much like homeopaths, consider such details as skin color, attitude, hair, nails, clothing, beliefs, and habits. In order for the cure to be complete, according to naturopaths, all potential problematic areas must be located and treated. Intensive personal interrogation is complex and often generates introspection about self, which has not previously been thought of as being important to health. We have provided a sample of the questions that will most likely be asked by a holistic naturopath.

The Naturopathic Exam

1. Do you enjoy your work?
2. How often do you bathe?
3. How do you describe yourself?
4. Do you listen to others' problems?
5. Are you affected by constraints on your time?
6. Do you have good lighting at home? At work?
7. Is the window open while you sleep?
8. How long do you sleep each day?
9. On what type of diet are you living? What types of foods are eaten most frequently?
10. How often do you eat? Do you relax during and after a meal?
11. How do you feel about yourself? Your future?
12. What bothers you about others?
13. In what type of environment do you live?
14. How do you feel immediately before symptoms of dis-ease appear?

Even though detail is also necessary in homeopathic examination, a healee is not classified according to symptoms in naturopathy, as is the case with homeopathy. Rather, naturopaths are of the opinion that an individual's dis-ease cannot be treated and/or cured by knowing symptoms alone; symptoms simply point out energy deficiencies. It then becomes the task of the naturopath to make use of all natural means "which have been found to affect the Vital Force beneficially in order that the self-repair processes of the body may be brought into action and relief and cure effected as early as possible" (Hewlett-Parsons, 1968). Although homeopaths and naturopaths may disagree on the specific value of symptomatology, we doubt that either would dispute the end result.

After examinations, practitioners individualize any natural measure deemed necessary to evoke the vital force to reestablish homeostatis. Many healing types are put to use simultaneously, or some may be utilized only once. In each case education occurs concurrently. We found that consumers help construct a program that will suit individual time schedules and needs. Practitioners, as a general rule, cleanse and nourish the system as a "first step" toward health. This, then, will be the beginning of a long and integrated plan to regain and preserve a dynamic balance between spirit, mind, and body. In most cases, cleansing and nourishing involves fasting on a few light foods and/or water for a period of three days. Blood, as the life stream of the body, must be purified and nourished to its optimum condition while the program is in effect, which, according to naturopaths, is imperative in a program of total health.

After cleansing has taken place, treatment is centered on rebuilding the body's strength. This is accomplished in a number of natural ways but begins with instruction about nutrition. Fresh foods are distinguished as primary nutritional recommendations. Additionally, practitioners stress that consumption of water helps rid the body of toxic wastes as well as fulfills one of the requirements of the influence of a natural element. Because of the influence of foods on bodily interactions, most patients are required to adhere to changes in diet during the treatment period. Practitioners organize and regulate food intake according to the quantity and quality of nutrients consumed and what is needed to initiate self-healing processes.

A consumer will most likely be prescribed some sort of medicament in the form of herbal teas, homeopathic substances, or botanical mixtures. These are employed for the express purpose of assisting the vital force through the energy contained in them. Some naturopaths declare vitamin supplementation as part of these corrective measures because of the biochemical reactions vitamins produce in the body. But, this is not a general belief held by all practitioners. Internal remedies are usually available for purchase from the healer's own pharmaceutical supply, are inexpensive, and relieve the consumer from a trip to a drug store.

There is a major benefit of naturopathy that stands out above all others. These healers educate consumers about every treatment method to be used. This not only includes the healing process, but side effects, virtues, why it is used, and how to adapt treatment(s) to home use. Previous patients of naturopaths highly praise the practitioners and methods of treatment. They report that personal care by the healer and his or her staff served to broaden their perspective about health. They also say that they learned about so many different areas that they felt "part of health" rather than sickness.

A naturopath, by definition, treats the whole person by exciting the self-healing functions inherent in the body. A healer assumes the responsibility for teaching one how to live, for restoring the body, and for relieving symptoms, but the consumer must make a commitment to health. You, then, must take the ultimate responsibility for decoding the underlying conflicting areas that create dis-ease and take steps toward the promotion of integrating mind, body, and spirit.

Diseases Treated

Naturopaths feel that they have been trained to treat, by natural measures, any and all dis-eases dealt with by scientifically trained general practitioners in the fields of family, community, and individual medicine. Naturopaths do not often perform major surgery. Since naturopaths maintain that they are knowledgeable in both scientific and natural methodologies, they purport that naturopathic medicine has combined knowledge of natural laws and scientific research (on individual methods, not naturopathy as a whole system) to activate self-healing functions in order to promote homeostasis.

Duration of Treatment

As intimated throughout this chapter, naturopathic healing is both costly and time consuming. Perhaps "time consuming" is an understatement. If one is in need of all or even half the treatments available, it is feasible that treatment can take six months of regular visits to resolve a health problem partially. Not all practitioners will use the many varieties of treatments available for each dis-ease, but those who employ only botanicals or homeopathic remedies to relieve symptoms are not considered true naturopaths by the majority of professionals in the field.

A patient who assumes that once overt symptoms have disappeared he or she is cured is simply operating upon incorrect assumptions. Reaching a balanced state in body, spirit, and mind involves many slow changes. According to practitioners, with each visit, outlined changes and their effects are assessed, discussed, and altered. Not until it is felt by both the healee and the practitioner that one has the knowledge, will, commitment, and means to health is one "officially" released from naturopathic care. Although treatments for symptoms may not take longer than two weeks or a month, practitioners report that counseling, restructuring, and instruction can take as long as a year.

Cost Range

The fees of naturopaths vary considerably, but most professionals charge a set fee that includes various treatments and counseling. Testing and pharmaceuticals are extra.

Initial visit—$20–$35 (Some adjust fees on a sliding-scale basis.)
Follow-up visit—$15–$30 (This fee is also adjustable.)
Testing—$125–$170 (This can be reduced by using a health clinic.)
Pharmaceuticals—$.75–$10

Personal Responsibilities

While reading this book, we hope that consumers become aware of the enormous responsibility placed upon them for the healing process and for implementing the holistic measures learned at home. One who employs a naturopathic healer must assume the maximum amount of responsibility in time and money in order to accomplish care of spirit, mind, and body. Additionally, faith in the practitioner, the natural methods, and the body's inherent healing ability is needed to assure a cure.

It is important that you realize the variation of possible treatments that may be used to heal dis-ease and restore health. It is unfair to expect a physician just to "relieve the symptoms." Naturopaths expect you to help design a detailed program of action for both cure of dis-ease and maintenance of optimum health in everyday life. The disease, you are told, can possibly return if all facets of the individual are not balanced to achieve homeostasis. Balance is a fluid process between body, mind, and spirit that aids individual regulation within the environment.

Consumers should question the healer about all diagnoses of dis-ease and treatments to be given. In many cases, your questions can accentuate the reliability of the process and provide more personal security and commitment to health. Questioning also reiterates interest in health by showing that you desire to learn the best means for achieving well-being. Furthermore, treatment measures within the healing setting provide necessary skills for implementation of them at home. Consumers must be sure that procedures are fully understood.

As we pointed out earlier, it may be difficult to discover the source of dis-ease unless one is willing to "open up" to the practitioner. Through education and counseling, the healee's personal feelings are intensely examined so that the major conflicts that surround lack of health can be dissolved. This process is a long and arduous one that involves mental stamina, durability, and will power. You must remember that all methods in holism are personally oriented. Practitioners do not judge reasons or actions. Instead, they help clients understand how particular reasoning and/or acts relate to dis-ease and how to change them for beneficial results.

If you do not wish to take part in a particular therapy, tell the healer. There are a number of overlapping beneficial therapies that can end in the same result. This also applies when you are unsure about procedure. Although all the therapies are explained before you participate, there may be a question in mind which causes a problem. It is best to ask the question when it comes to mind rather than inhibiting it. Inhibition of a doubt, no matter how small, can stagnate the reception of energy from that particular method. According to healers, this in effect blocks the beneficial effect on the vital force.

Last, thoroughly check on your physician's reliability with other patients. We found that many who listed a D.C., N.D. combination after their name often placed more emphasis on chiropractic methods. Most holistic practitioners will gladly provide you with names of healees who have received treatment. For the most part you can resolve any conflict by simply questioning those in the waiting room. This is important because of the lack of general published information about naturopathy as a healing system. Since the methods have not been proven experimentally in their entirety, you will have to become familiar with enough material to make decisions on each segment of the treatment. Do not forget to check on the licensing requirements for naturopaths within your state.

Remember that naturopaths assume that the vital force contained within each human being initiates the healing process. You must have faith in the existence and ability of the vital force to "duplicate" the healthy state or you may be wasting your time. If you are too cynical or skeptical about this belief, you should seek care elsewhere. The vital force, a link between the cosmos and the everyday world, is intangible. Yet faith accompanies all healing processes. In holistic methods, faith in the cure is an integral part of success in healing.

Informational Organizations

National College of Naturopathic Medicine
501 S.W. Third Avenue, Room 415
Portland, OR 97204

National Association of Naturopathic Physicians
PO Box 1648
609 Sherman Avenue
Coeur d'Alene, ID 83814

American Association of Constitutional Medicine
405 Appleway Avenue
Coeur d'Alene, ID 83813

There are some state organizations that can aid consumers in locating practitioners in their specific areas. These organizations also disseminate a limited amount of information about naturopathy. Addresses for state associations are in the yellow pages of telephone directories in the following states: Alabama, District of Columbia, Florida, Idaho, Indiana, Kansas, Louisiana, Michigan, Montana, North Carolina, Ohio, Oregon, Texas, Utah, and Washington. Occasionally, chiropractors may also know of practitioners in naturopathy.

Consistencies

1. The definition of naturopathy encompasses the healing of physical, mental, spiritual, and environmental levels of the individual. It is the goal of naturopathy to teach one how to maintain harmony within a total life environment.

2. Naturopathic physicians are vitally aware that each individual is unique and requires matchless treatment. They also assume that responsibility for a disorder resides with the individual.

3. Only natural substances are used as medicaments. Less expensive, naturopaths point out that remedies are as reliable as man-made pharmaceuticals that were originally derived from these very substances. Natural medicaments must adhere to natural laws before they are put to use.

4. Practitioners employ any natural method needed to treat dis-ease. The multidimensional nature of this modality thereby qualifies it as being consistent with the holistic philosophy.

5. Individualized nutritional considerations and exercise are two immediate actions taken by these healers. Healees are urged to give the wholesome basics an intimate place in their environment and encompass exercise techniques into their daily lives.

6. A client is expected to be an equal partner in diagnosis and treatment of dis-ease. This not only involves receiving treatment but includes the healee working in an alliance to establish a program suitable for maintaining well-being after treatment.

7. The spiritual element, made of vibrations within the vital force, is linked to the basis of the universe. Natural methods and medicaments are based on the laws of nature to reestablish homeostasis, the body's natural healing process.

8. Educational instruction provides consumers with an understanding of dis-ease and its interrelationship to self, nature, and science. Teaching strategies include promotion of health, self-care, and maintenance of health.

Inconsistencies

1. Naturopathy establishes the fact that all diseases are treatable by this method in spite of its practitioners' lack of "orthodox" scientific training in medicine. Practitioners train as general physicians. Most other holistic modes are as specialized as formal medicine, whereas naturopathy includes all specialties.

2. Practitioners in most other holistic fields do not dare compare themselves to physicians for fear of prosecution, whereas naturopaths do. Naturopaths give diagnoses and treatment which may result in legal problems in some states.

3. The use of electricity can be very dangerous. Even though justifications that electricity and electromagnetic energy have similar properties, we found few other holistic practices that make use of electricity.

4. Naturopathy seems to be the "allopathy" of holism in that these practitioners are formally trained in both scientific and naturalistic treatment methods for all dis-eases and combine both indoctrinations to cure and prevent dis-ease.

5. The existence of the vital force must be accepted on grounds of faith. However, science itself has based its empirical studies on faith.

6. Why is naturopathy restricted by state laws which either limit or disallow its use if, in fact, it has successfully cured so many? Why is there no published evidence about its effectiveness as a *total system* of healing? It seems that practitioners have relied upon previous research in varied individual natural methods for its scientific credence.

7. Unlike other holistic measures, naturopathy is expensive simply because of the time required to procure a "total cure," as defined by naturopathic healers. Thus, the holistic procedure will not reduce treatment costs. However, learning preventive measures will tend to decrease future medical costs.

8. In naturopathy, the consumer goes through extensive reeducation for self-healing, whereas other holistic modalities do not require so much in order to provide the consumer with home health measures.

Sources to Read

Abbot, A. E., ed. *The Art of Healing.* London: Emerson Press, 1963.

Airola, Paavo. *How to Get Well.* Phoenix, AZ: Health Press Publishers, 1974.

Anderson, Mary. *Colour Healing.* New York: Weiser, 1975.

Benjamin, Harry. *Everybody's Guide to Nature Cure.* New York: British Book Center, 1976.

Berren, Faber. *Light, Color and Environment.* New York: Van Nostrand Reinhold, 1969.

Bieler, Henry G. *Food Is Your Best Medicine.* New York: Random House, 1965.

Bricklin, Mark. *The Practical Encyclopedia of Natural Healing.* Emmaus, PA: Rodale Press, 1976.

Clark, Linda. *Ancient Art of Color Therapy.* Old Greenwich, CT: Devin-Adair, 1975.

Clements, G. R. *The Law of Life and Human Health.* Mokelumne Hill, CA: Health Research, 1972.

Clymer, R. S. *The Natural Physician.* Quakertown, PA: Philosophical Publishing Co., 1933.

Devi, Indra. *Forever Young, Forever Healthy.* New York: Arco, 1953.

Ehret, Arnold. *Rational Fasting.* New York: Benedict Lust, 1974.

Gandhi, Mohandas K. *Nature Cure.* Bombay: Bharatiya Vidya Bhavan, 1966.

Garten, M. O. *The Health Secrets of a Naturopathic Doctor.* Englewood Cliffs, NJ: Prentice Hall, 1967.

————. *The Natural and Drugless Way for Better Health.* New York: Arc Books, 1971.

Hewlett-Parsons, J., D.Sc. *Naturopathic Practice.* New York: Arco, 1968.

Jackson, Mildred, and **Teague, T.** *Handbook of Alternatives to Chemical Medicine.* Oakland, CA: Lawton-Teague Publishers, 1975.

Jennings, Charles. "Naturopathy," in *Well Being Magazine.* No. 24, Los Angeles, CA: 1979, pp. 17–22.

Jensen, Bernard. *You Can Master Disease.* Bolana Beach, CA: Bernard Jensen, 1952.

Just, Adolf. *Return to Nature.* Mokelumne Hill, CA: Health Research, 1970.

Kulvinskas, Viktoras. *Survival into the Twenty-First Century.* Wethersfield, CT: Omangod Press, 1975.

Moyle, Alan. *Natural Health for the Elderly.* Northants, England: Thorsons, 1975.

National College of Naturopathic Medicine *Bulletin*, 1981–82.

Newman, Laura, M.D. *Make Your Juicer Your Own Drug Store.* Simi Valley, CA: Benedict Lust, 1972.

Poesnecker, G.E. *The Clymer Health Clinic: It's Only Natural.* Lansdale, PA: Ad Venturia, 1975.

Powell, Eric. *Natural Home Physician.* Rustington, Sussex, England: Health Science Press, 1975.

Roberts, Jane. *The Nature of Personal Reality.* Englewood Cliffs, NJ: Prentice-Hall, 1976.

Spitler, Harry R. *Basic Naturopathy.* Columbus, OH: American Naturopathic Association, 1948.

Tribe, Bill. "Naturopathic Medicine," in *Holistic Health Handbook.* Edward Brint, et. al. Berkeley, CA: And/Or Press, 1978.

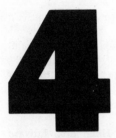

HOMOEOPATHY

Definition

Homoeopathy is another method of healing that evolved from the statements of Hippocrates. He said, "Through the like, disease is produced and through the application of the like it is cured" (Vargo, n.d.). Hippocrates felt that the *theory of similia*, a law he considered natural, could best affect the symptoms of disease by making use of a small amount of a substance that produces an approximation of the patient's disorder. Paracelsus added to Hippocrates' theory by pointing out that physicians should make use of intuition in diagnosing and treating dis-ease and that the underlying causes of dis-ease could be based upon mental and/or emotional factors. Furthermore, Paracelsus felt that symptoms were a reflection of the dis-ease, but that the source could only be found by examining the whole person (Mitchell, 1975).

Samuel Hahnemann, a German physician who had studied in orthodox medical establishments of the time, took note of the fact that medicine did not "cure" many of his patients. What was called an "ancient" theory, *the law of similars*, had once been employed by Hindu sages and Chinese practitioners to treat disorders that were not responding to the medicinal procedures of the time. While researching the theory of similars, Hahnemann discovered that Hippocrates and Paracelsus successfully treated patients using this theory. Further exploration led Hahnemann to one of the fundamental principles of the natural sciences (physics, chemistry, biology, and physiology) expressing the idea that any agitation in equilibrium will eventually produce circumstances returning equilibrium. Within medicine, this became known as *homeostasis*.

Hahnemann began experimenting with the self-healing abilities of the body in conjunction with the use of drugs that produced reactions similar to those the patient was experiencing. Later, physiologist Rudolph Arndt proved that chemical reactions could be affected by dosages of specific amounts. Arndt demonstrated that:

1. Small substances excite reactions.
2. Medium doses favor reactions.
3. Large doses dull or stop reactions.

In the 1880's another researcher, Hugo Schulz, applied Arndt's findings to medicine and revolutionized the field with the Arndt-Schulz Law.

Years earlier, Hahnemann, with similar ideas of dosage quantity and reactions in mind, experimented on himself with a tree bark reported to cure a fever. He found that the tree bark did indeed induce the same symptoms as the fever. Decreasing the dosage with each new experiment, Hahnemann slowly collected evidence by recording the symptoms and changes in his mental, physical, and emotional state. After each smaller dose, the "cure" became more rapid, just as the Arndt-Schulz law later predicted. Thus, the law of similars worked on Hahnemann.

In order for a disabled body to reach homeostasis, Hahnemann believed, the vital forces of the body would have to be excited by the small dose of the curative agent. To this end he invented a method called *succession* for releasing a curative's vital energies. In this method, the latent medicinal properties of crude substances are made dynamic so that they directly attend to the vital forces within the body. He felt that infinitesimal doses of the *one* correct substance would allow the vital forces to attack a minute form of the illness. By attacking this illness on a cellular level, the vital forces would thereby destroy the "real" dis-ease using these same defenses, much like inoculations protect us from such dis-eases as polio today. The theory of homoeopathy is based upon four major practical principles. They are as follows:

1. Substances which produce the same symptoms like an individual is experiencing will cure that individual. This is called the *law of similars*.
2. Only one dose is needed.
3. A minimum, successed dosage is most potent.
4. In order to attain homeostasis, vital forces, which are dynamic, must also be set into motion by the individual.

In the late 1700s and early 1800s homoeopathy became extremely popular with physicians and clients alike. Hahnemann's methods were practiced throughout Europe and in the U.S., where, according to homoeopathic research, practitioners cured cholera, typhoid, scarlet fever, smallpox, and other disorders when orthodox physicians and techniques failed.

When some of the orthodox physicians moved to have homoeopathy absorbed into the AMA, the debating that took place between allopathic and homoeopathic physicians was bitter. Colleges fought colleges; hospitals split their affiliations and refused to set up practice rooms for homoeopathic or orthodox practitioners; orthodox physicians would not be in the same room with homoeopaths. The medical profession was extremely divided and Hahnemann did not help matters. He publicly stated that drugs used by orthodox doctors were prescribed on the basis of opposite reactions to symptoms, which violated natural laws. In fact, it was Hahnemann who originally termed orthodox practitioners "allopaths," meaning treatments "opposite from suffering." This was deeply resented by most physicians because it insinuated that allopaths practiced with any theory in order to cure disease. (Kaufman, 1971; Mitchell, 1975).

One of the first actions of the newly formed American Medical Association was to formulate the consultation clause in their Code of Ethics in 1847. The clause prohibited consultations between physicians if one was orthodox and one was "sectarian," such as homoeopathy. In fact, Kaufman asserts that the struggle against homoeopathy was a major factor in the formation of the AMA (Kaufman, 1971, pp. 52–54). After being barred from the AMA, homoeopathy later gained respectability and was accepted or absorbed by the AMA in 1903. After that, this school of medicine declined until the birth of the holistic health movement. Some experts have attributed the decline of homoeopathy directly to its absorption by orthodox medicine (Kaufman, 1971, p. 173).

Currently, the National Center for Homoeopathy defines homoeopathy as "a system of drug treatment for sick people (not diseases) which is based on the Law of Similars, the minimum dose and the single remedy proven on human beings." It is an individualized process that combines science and art to treat dis-ease, excite self-healing processes, and dissolve the source(s) of disorders. Homoeopathy supposedly treats the whole person: mental/emotional and physical relationships to dis-ease. Practitioners must obtain a composite symptomatology in order to prescribe one minimum, potent dose.

Presently, licensed health care professionals can only seek post-graduate training in the field. That is, after official training is com-pleted, interested *physicians* (and selected others in health care) study homoeopathy. The curriculum involves history, workings of the laws of nature, research, the study of symptoms, homoeotherapeutics, mental/emotional factors relating to dis-ease, and prescription of dosages. No degree or certification (except a certificate of attendance) can be given. However, they have filed an application with the AMA to be able to give continuing education credit for the work but have not yet received formal permission. The limited few that hold the coveted D-HT were awarded the title by the American Board of Homoeotherapeutics for outstanding contributions to the field or have studied outside of the U.S. and were certified there. Homoeopaths make use of a vast array of intellectual and intuitive facts learned from both the allopathic and homoeopathic schools of medicine which are united in their practice. G. Rughven Mitchell stated in this book *Homeopathy* (1975) "although in perhaps ninety percent of cases homeopathy will prove self-sufficient, for the remainder he (physician) will apply allopathic methods, either alone or in conjunction with his own remedies."

The healee is most influential to the success of a cure. The precise dosage for treatment is dependent upon the healee's detailed description of his or her symptoms, termed "generals." In homoeopathic diagnosis there are physical "generals," mental "generals," and modifying or changing factors in addition to rare, strange, or peculiar indications practitioners have named "particulars." Homoeopaths compile a dis-tinct composite of signs that allows him or her to individualize the remedy to "fit" *all* signs of the dis-ease as expressed by the patient.

Homoeopaths differ from other healers in that they must find *one* substance to match all symptoms of the disorder at that point in time *exactly*. Their observations, then, must be highly individualized in order for a thorough description of symptoms to be completed. You will remember Hahnemann's fourth principle in Homoeopathy states ex-plicitly that the individual must aid in the healing process by awaken-ing his or her own vital forces. The integration of the client into the healing process is accomplished by involving the healee in diagnosis and treatment processes as well as individualized education in maintain-ing well-being. Practitioner and client work as a team in order to find the correct dosage, pinpoint problematic beliefs and habits, and change facets that inhibit an individual's self-regulating powers. This cannot be accomplished by a healer alone; thus, one who chooses this method must be prepared for extended visitations.

Education for healees is individualized and is given during the period of treatment. Nutrition, life-style habits, relaxation and stress reduction, and exercise are integral components of homoeopathic teachings. Each of these is reorganized or restructed to promote total health. Homoeopaths consider their field as "distinct from Holistic Medicine yet exemplifying its pure essence" (National Center for Homoeopathy, 1980). A major focus of the learning process is acknowledging that multiple factors relate to health and, more importantly, that each person contains inherent capabilities for health and harmony.

The major controversy remaining in homoeopathy today is over the "dynamized" infinitesimal dosage used to awaken the vital force. It was Hahnemann's belief that the drug must be dynamized to activate the spirit of the substance. Practitioners affirm that any remedy employed for treatment in homoeopathy has multiple functions in that it affects all levels of the ailment. In addition, each must go through experimental testing before it is considered for use on patients. The total symptomatology of the substance is listed in the *Homoeopathic Materia Medica*, which is a list of facts and symptoms characteristic of the essences employed by homoeopaths. Because of the importance of homoeopathic prescription, we will provide a more lengthy discussion of the experimental procedure conducted on potential remedies in the next section of this chapter.

Homoeopathy encompasses holism without defining itself as holistic. Rather, practitioners consider homoeopathy as a distinct art and science, a system unique to any other. Homoeopaths believe that they promote balance and harmony within the individual by making use of the accumulation of scientific evidence and natural laws.

Many vitalists believe that they have verified the existence of the vital force as the essence of all living things and the power to heal the self, homeostasis. Homoeopathy asserts these same beliefs are in accordance with a holistic viewpoint. They propose that treatment of body, mind, and emotions are necessary links for curing dis-ease and promoting well-being. Dis-ease is dynamic in cause and nature and, therefore, must be treated by dynamic dosage. Ease is also dynamic and must be constructed by integrating and acting upon those factors that prove to be deteriorating to the dynamic balance of the vital force.

Type of Healing

To be completely objective, homoeopathy cannot be considered a totally natural method, even though many of its foundations, laws, and concepts are natural. There is one major reason behind this statement. By its own admission and by definition, practitioners must be licensed medical doctors who have been trained in scientific medicine and taught to reject natural laws in favor of scientific ones. On the other hand, these scientific procedures lend credence to the natural laws of cure upon which homoeopathy is based. Homoeopathy, therefore, straddles the gap between natural healing methods and scientific procedure. Previous clients that we interviewed were unable to classify homoeopathy as a totally natural method, even though practitioners reportedly employed only natural remedies and techniques. They also told us that they "felt" like practitioners were physicians and some were even diagnosed and treated by means of the computer. Medicaments were also, according to healees, another reason homoeopathy seemed more medical than natural.

Theoretically, the diluted small dose decreases the cells' sensitivity to dis-ease by providing the cell with the opportunity to construct natural barriers against the disorder by way of the vital force. Nerve fibers detect the presence of the remedy and impulses move throughout the body. Some practitioners state that nerve reaction is all that is needed to excite the body's recuperative abilities. Others feel that the substance alters cell membranes and influences enzymes igniting the vital forces through enzyme performance. Regardless of practitioners' scientific explanations, the initiation of the life force is the purpose of a dynamized remedy.

Homoeopathic literature is adamant about remedies being proven on the healthy human being. The experimental scheme is much more extensive than case study procedures offered as proof in some of the other holistic fields. Called the double-blind method, a voluntary "prover" is given a purified, refined, successed substance, or a placebo, by an expert administer. Neither the "prover" nor the "expert" knows if the substance is a drug or not until after the "proving" is completed. Vibrational and emotional relations, just as physical ones, are given equal importance in the analysis of the drug by both the expert and the prover. Every possible character, reaction, localization, and action is recorded for future reference to enable a practitioner to match the exact symptomatology of an individual. Curatives similar in "vibration" to the nature of the dis-ease are important because they "match" the unique pulsation of the disorder and the vital force. In light of the fact that orthodox medical research, as we know it and according to practitioners, tests drugs on rabbits, monkeys, cats, rats, guinea pigs, or other animals, it seems that homoeopathy exceeds their requirements.

The American Institute of Homoeopathy maintains that conclusive scientific evidence, using double-blind procedures, has already been published by several foreign researchers (Koetschan; Beir and Landel; Schoeler; Nettier; Persson; Boyd; Robilliart and Lesser; and Janner) substantiating the unquestionable effectiveness of the small, potentized dosage employed by homoeopaths. These researchers argue that the Arndt-Schulz law demonstrates the characteristics and applicability of small doses, whereas the dynamic nature of dis-ease justifies the procedure of succession to excite a substance's vital essences. According to this research, homoeopathic remedies do not offer prolonged side effects and are most effective for those with allergic reactions.

Homoeopaths boast that their drugs produce no side effects because of the extensive experimental procedures they have undergone before they are admitted to the *Materia Medica*. Yet our research tells us that a number of reactions often occur when the dosage is consumed. Symptoms may tend to feel exaggerated or stronger or one may experience profuse sweating, diarrhea, skin eruptions, and other effects. Practitioners explain that these responses are only temporary and that they indicate the correct substance was prescribed. The body's vital forces have been activated by the drug.

Homoeopaths further instruct patients to look for signs of healing. They point out that healing, in most cases, takes place in four general ways. They are:

1. From above downward: Headache disappears and soreness in legs appears.
2. From inside to outside: Nausea disappears and a cold sore appears.
3. From vital to less vital organs: Pain around the heart disappears and a bladder infection appears.
4. In reverse order: Symptoms appearing last disappear first.

Since reactions are individualized this information should prepare one for what may take place. This is not, by any means, always the way homoeopathic treatment works.

The fact that Hahnemann recommended *one* small, excited substance to affect the dynamic forces in the individual seems somewhat ambiguous. Most practitioners are known to employ more than one drug even though these may be given during separate visitations. According to healers in this field one may require a remedy for each set of symptoms in order to rebuild the body and to aid the body's recuperative powers. In most cases, it is unlikely that one dose will completely cure symptoms, although that is preferred.

There are two contradictory characteristics that are apparent in homoeopathy. One of these is that little orientation is provided for preventing dis-ease, even though it can, supposedly, prevent dis-ease. When compared with naturopathy or even nutritional therapy, homoeopathy is severely lacking in this area. Although some educational instruction is provided during an individual treatment period, most of it is focused on mental awareness and acknowledgment of the problem rather than techniques for preventing reccurrences. Generally, there is no program designed by the healee and physician to maintain health. There is an obvious difference between *telling* one about the sources of a disorder versus construction of *acts* that will prevent the disorder.

Another contradiction is that practitioners will work with orthodox physicians only under certain conditions. Healers point out that homoeopathy is more effective with surgery and/or specialized care, whereas treatment has limited effects for those already receiving medication, antibiotics, sulfa, or steroids. On the other hand, homoeotherapeutics is suitable with nutritional therapy, endocrine therapy, obstetrics, psychology and psychiatry, osteopathy, physical therapy, naturopathy, and chiropractic (Baker, 1977). It appears that homoeopathy is all things to all people.

An outstanding attribute of homoeopathy is that practitioners are always willing to share information, to explain the practice, or to answer a question for consumers. We found that homoeopaths and their professional associations are most cooperative in providing impartial information to consumers about this method. It is their aim to destroy the myths surrounding the art-science and to promote homoeopathy as a viable method of healing. The propulsive qualities of dis-ease and pharmaceuticals have created a medical structure that converges naturalism/vitalism with science. To the consumer who wishes the security of orthodox medical science and the fundamentals of natural therapy, homoeopathy is the ideal medical system. Mental-emotional interrelations are the distinctive focal points within treatment of the whole person. Healers, by choice, prepare the healee for the actions that accompany health, but once the consumer is cognizant of unhealthy mental-emotional patterns, he or she must assume absolute responsibility for promoting healthful changes.

Description of Healing Method

The consumer who decides to try homoeopathic treatment is usually advised to have chemical testing (hair, urine, and blood) completed before visiting a practitioner. Though homoeopaths perform a general physical examination, X rays, and a detailed case history, most healers do not have the required equipment for laboratory analysis. A public health clinic or a specialist can provide access to these tests at an extra expense. Though this may seem burdensome, remember that they are trained physicians as well as homoeopaths and do not forsake the allopathic aspects of the healing profession.

Because of the itemized indications that make up a composite representing the dis-ease and the individual, a first trip to this practitioner should take hours. Some healees have reported talking with a practitioner for as long as four hours as well as "waiting hours for him to decide which drug was best" for activation of the life forces.

The case-taking method is time consuming because of the details the healee is required to contribute during diagnosis. We thought readers would be interested in a glimpse of some questions and descriptions one faces during diagnosis by a homoeopath. A selection of these follows:

Descriptions and Questions Concerning Symptoms

1. How did your problem begin and how has it changed?
2. Previous illnesses, locations, and treatments?
3. Describe your nervous and mental problems.
4. How is your appetite? What do you eat? What time do you eat?
5. Are you thirsty? When? How much and what do you drink each day?
6. Describe your pain. Location? How long has it hurt? What time does it hurt most?
7. Which season are you functioning best? Worst?
8. What conditions make you better or worse?
9. Are you affected by the weather? How?
10. Do your symptoms remain the same or change? How do they change?
11. What are your cravings? Dislikes?
12. How do you feel about your future? What do you do for relaxation?
13. How do you feel about failure? Do you like your job?
14. How are you affected by those around you? At work? Other friends?

Additionally there are an extensive number of questions concerning sensations, skin, discharges, urine, bowels, and male and female problems. This is just a small sample of the minute characteristics needed by a healer at the time of examination.

We should note that strange or peculiar signs of diseases are important for an accurate diagnosis. Often it is these symptoms that distinguish a particular drug that will activate the vital forces. As explained earlier, homoeopaths take into account how symptoms distinguish themselves but they are more concerned with "generals" for description of disorders. As one can see by the list of questions just provided, "generals" describe the total individual. Because a healee's mental-emotional views are current indications of dis-ease, the consumer will have to be introspective for this healing mode. All case-taking and symptoms name the illness, describe a healee's unique nature, and point to a remedy to aid the natural process of homeostasis.

By using the detailed "holistic" history, the practitioner must individualize the patient's inventory and description of symptoms. He or she evaluates symptoms by considering severity, time present, localization, and character in order to determine if the person can be cured through homoeopathic treatment. Remember that homoeopathy attends sick *persons*, not *dis-eases*. In short, the healer must decide if the dis-ease will respond to homoeopathic treatment, given the personal characteristics of an individual. He or she will then index symptoms so as to provide dosages that produce the *exact* symptoms of the dis-ease as characterized by both healee and practitioner. The healer will likely consult the Homoeopathic Materia Medica, which lists facts and symptoms about drugs, to determine the minimal substance that will excite the vital forces toward homeostatic growth. The remedy chosen will match the totality of one's symptoms in physical, mental, and emotional areas.

Most homoeopathic physicians prefer to see clients at least three times. If one's disorder is complicated and extremely serious, the number of visits increases to as many as twenty-four. And, here is another discrepancy within homoeopathy. Homoeopaths believe that one dose of a highly potentized substance initiates the self-healing processes by exciting the vital force. Yet, a serious dis-ease, (and most others for that matter) may require more than one homoeopathic remedy. In fact, we have talked with several healees who were given one or more doses over a designated time, even though this is taboo in the homoeopathic philosophy. As consumers, many of us think that drugs prescribed over a period of time is a natural procedure. But within homoeopathy this is a critical point that is only partially explained by practitioners in the field. The majority of healers feel that more than one dose *is not true homoeopathy*, but also point out that other doses may be necessary in order to assure that one is healed. We reconcile the difference by deciding that practitioners have left this point purposefully vague in order to meet the demands of extreme cases, complicated disorders, and certain individuals.

Most consumers find a trip into the world of homoeopathy very enlightening. The healee is taught that homeostasis is the body's regulating device. If one part of the system malfunctions, it affects all other parts of the regulator. Although the regulator (homeostasis) should adjust itself, it frequently requires aid. The healee becomes aware of a multitude of links that stir both vitality and sickness. Consumers report being continually amazed when healers lead them to see the factors influencing health and dis-ease and that homoeopathic treatment provides a kind of "private cartharsis" for the healee. Although the educational procedure is limited to counseling techniques, it seems that this has been sufficient in producing life-style, belief, and nutritional changes for most of the healees we have interviewed. In order to prevent dis-ease and maintain homeostasis, a healee procures intuitive understanding of health through the homoeopath but acquires more practical knowledge on his or her own. Therefore, the patient assumes most of the responsibility for upkeep of health and interception of dis-ease.

Diseases Treated

Hahnemann's philosophy espouses that dis-ease is dynamic. Accordingly, homoeopathy will treat any dis-ease with the dynamized dose. However, we do not wish to project false hopes. The homoeopath can finely tune a body, but a truly healthy state is composed of personal concern for and action toward flexible relationships among emotional, mental, and physical factors in order to attain homeostasis. According to practicing homoeopaths, these must be acquired by the healee over a period of time and, in most cases, they require definite changes in daily habits.

Although all types of dis-eases are treated by homoeopaths, we found evidence supporting cures for the following: asthma, influenza viruses, epilepsy, such mental disorders as depression and anxiety, bronchitis, infantile dis-ease, infectious diseases, arthritis, bursitis, kidney stones and infections, cold sores, varicose veins, irregular heartbeat, heart disease, sinusitus, eye disorders, skin eruptions, ulcers, tumors, insomnia, allergies, syphilis, urinary and bladder inflections, prostate disorders, female problems, gallbladder disorders, gallstones, and most nervous or nerve-related conditions. Homoeopathy does not claim to cure dis-eases in cases of physical malformation, tissue damage, advanced cancer, or where major surgery is indicated.

Duration of Treatment

The number of visitations with a homoeopath is based upon the changes that may or may not have occurred from the original minimum dose treatment and the severity of the dis-ease. If the infinitesimal remedy has awakened innate healing ability and excited the vital forces in such a way that the disorder is moving out of the system, then treatment is relatively short. Equally important to practitioners is individual progress toward the absorption and implementation of recommended changes in nutrition, life-style, and mental-emotional interaction, which the healee has experienced during diagnosis and treatment. This aspect of homoeopathic treatment often necessitates more time because of the fundamental alterations that take place in personal awareness.

Actual office visitations with a practitioner average about six for most dis-eases. Some previous patients report continued treatment for as many as twenty-four separate consultations. However, these former healees point out that it was their choice to continue for much of that period. Interestingly, we found that most were completely cured of their symptoms. Healees must report changes in physical and mental-emotional condition with each visit. The demand for patient involvement is such that if one does not develop in the direction of total well-being, treatment must be extended.

Cost Range

Initial visit—$12–$25
Follow-up visit—$10–$15
Counseling—included with visit
Lay Courses—$25 and up
Prescriptions—$.75 and up (many are included with physician fee)

Practitioners often adjust fees on a sliding scale basis to accommodate those who are unable to pay or those who are on tight budgets.

Personal Responsibilities

Perhaps the most distinctive consumer responsibility is the understanding of the theory underlying homoeopathy. We suggest writing the National Center for Homoeopathy for brochures on the subject or reading one of the books listed in the references at the end of the chapter. Personal understanding of homoeopathy prevents expectations of a fast, quick-acting cure. Advanced knowledge enhances this method by preparing one for the type of treatment modality, the philosophical basis, the time involved, and the problems one may encounter.

Many practitioners of homoeopathy may be licensed health professionals, but not physicians. Some have apprenticed under doctors, some have studied but have not been given certification of that fact, and others have attended postgraduate training. Each of these practitioners have "healed" those who recommended them to us by making use of homoeopathy. But, because of the lay network of homoeopathy and the fact that lay practitioners do not have to be physicians, we urge that one be very careful when selecting a practitioner for treatment. On the other hand, a physician with a D-HT degree, and there are very few, does not necessarily make the best practitioner. Learn enough about homoeopathy in advance to know if a healer is being consistent with the holistic philosophy. Research the practitioner and his or her cures and talk with patients. If a healer refuses to let you call or talk with former clients, find another.

If you have recently had required testing for allopathic treatment, be sure to tell the practitioner ahead of time so that he or she will not waste time on it. This type of advanced preparation can save you both valuable treatment time. If you are taking drugs based upon an allopathic diagnosis, you will be required to discontinue all medication when you are undergoing homoeopathic treatment. Since most homoeopaths are physicians, they will want a complete history of previous treatment, especially if you are experiencing a chronic condition. If possible, obtain copies of an allopath's previous history for the practitioner. (Have the physician mail it directly to the homoeopath.) However, if you are being "treated" by a lay homoeopath, you are subscribing to an unlicensed lay person who does not possess the legitimate authority to diagnose and treat disease.

It is helpful to take some time to think about a dis-ease before one first visits the practitioner. While doing so, try to remember when it began, how it felt, how it changed, what was happening around you at the time, how long it has lasted, and any other details you may have observed, even if they seemed insignificant at the time. This process will help you when a description of symptoms is requested by the practitioner. As an equal partner in the diagnosis process, an accurate description of symptoms will help with the choice of the substance prescribed.

Dilution of a substance, homoeopaths tell us, allows the successed life force power of the dosage to scatter into a mixing solution, usually milk sugar or diluted alcohol. In other words, the drug's powers enter into the alcohol or milk sugar, giving not only more of something to take but also increasing the reaction of the small dosage on the body's vital forces. For this reason, remedies must be consumed with regularity.

One might speculate that the vital force is actually only an approximation of the natural immunizing properties of the body, but this has not yet been tested experimentally by homoeopaths. For information on this subject see Hans Selye (1979) and the Simontons (1978). Though still preliminary, this evidence does support homoeopathy's beliefs about the vital force, even though these theories differ in their explanations.

Although many may interpret this as a self-fulfilling prophecy, we suggest that anyone contemplating homoeopathic treatment be prepared for reaction to the minute dosage. Ask the healer to describe possible responses if he or she does not do this before a drug is consumed. Do not expect the drug to heal in ten minutes, and do not expect the cure to be a lasting one with transformations in other directions. The infinitesimal dose only activates the vital forces; the healee must complete the cure. A cure takes much longer than simply ridding the body of overt symptoms. The consumer interested in this field will have to be willing to take actions toward altering deleterious life-style habits and diet as well as some part of the daily routine.

Informational Organizations

International Homeopathic League
c/o Frederic W. Schmid, M.D., D-HT.
6200 Geary Boulevard
Medical Bldg. at 26th Avenue
San Francisco, CA 94121

Women's National Homeopathic League, Inc.
1911 Walnut Street
Dover, OH 44622

American Institute of Homoeopathy, Inc.
6231 Leesburg Pike, Suite 506
Falls Church, VA 22044

National Center for Homoeopathy
1500 Massachusetts Avenue, Suite 163
Washington, D.C. 20005

Consistencies

1. One of the major assumptions of homoeopathy is that the vital force residing within the body must be activated in order for treatment to be successful. This is in agreement with the holistic belief that the body contains the essential elements for preserving health and well-being. Whereas many vitalists believe in the existence of the vital force, and it is a common element in most of the fields in this book, the process of homeostasis, derived from the natural sciences, is a basic assumption of the scientific medical philosophy. One might further speculate that the vital force is actually only an approximation of the immunizing properties of the body often used by modern physicians to describe the significance of spontaneous remissions of such deadly diseases as cancer (Simonton and Simonton). Similar processes are occurring while the explanations of these differ.

2. Homoeopathic physicians treat the patient as an equal partner in the diagnosis process. This is partially a fundamental element of the holistic philosophy. After all, practitioners rely upon a person's description of their own symptoms before prescribing a substance designed to produce similar conditions. Finally, the counseling and education programs utilized within this type of treatment modality further emphasize this consistency, as do the more formal lay education programs.

3. In keeping with the principles of holism is the idea that a diagnosis must be made by collecting the totality of all the symptoms reported by the patient and observed by the practitioner. Healing also has to be total as it usually takes a longer duration of treatment. Though most of us have grown accustomed to fast recovery from specialists, homoeopathy emphasizes the whole person (mental, emotional, and physical), which consequently is more time consuming.

4. Homoeopathy has been found to be most effective when dealing with illnesses and sensitive or allergic patients. Research on the topic attributes this success to a thoroughly detailed diagnosis, the principle of like cures like, and mental and emotional changes by the healee. Additionally, all of the remedies prescribed by homoeopathic physicians have been "proven" on healthy people, as opposed to laboratory animals. These double-blind experiments wherein all characteristics and reactions are observed and recorded in both experimental and control groups lend extra credence to this modality.

5. Homoeopathy enjoys the position of being based upon natural laws and scientifically proven treatments. They can be acceptable, therefore, to scientists and lay persons alike. In this sense they enjoy the best of both worlds.

Inconsistencies

1. Though the definition of homoeopathy provides for the treatment of physical, mental, and emotional aspects of the person, spiritual, social, and environmental forces are noticeably absent from their definition. We wonder why they expanded physical characteristics, the sole focus of orthodox medicine, and omit these other levels. This is a major discrepancy because in order for a healing method to be holistic, spiritual concerns as well as environmental and social ones must be included as vital areas for treatment. One possible explanation for this omission is the fact that most homoeopaths are licensed physicians and they may have found that the more controversial realms of social, environmental, and spiritual problems are best left to others.

2. While placing a great deal of emphasis upon facilitating the patient's own healing processes and consumer education, they neglect the fact that the natural abilities of the body may not always need classical drug treatment. Therefore, they overemphasize the dependence of patients upon the treatment process rather than focusing upon promotion of health maintenance. To this extent, homoeopaths still rely upon the medical model rather than a holistic approach. While they emphasize that they are holistic, they do not stress life-style change to the extent of other holistic methods.

3. When compared with nutritional therapy or naturopathy, homoeopathy is severely limiting its scope by the omission of prevention and health-sustaining techniques. While some education and counseling occurs, there is no program of total health promotion designed for the consumer in consultation with the healer. As we mentioned earlier, there is a definite difference between telling one the underlying sources of the symptoms and facilitating changes in order to maintain health and prevent dis-ease before it develops.

4. While what we are about to describe is not inconsistent with holism, it is a basic contradiction in professional certification. Homoeopathy can only be studied in postgraduate courses and the D-HT is given to relatively few physicians with no distinct formal requirements. Though this is due in part to the political dominance of allopaths, it still leaves the consumer with an ambiguous definition of certified homoeopaths and denies the affirmation by these practitioners that they are a medical specialty.

5. A further inconsistency involves the contradiction between what the promotional literature emphasizes about homoeopathy and the actual experience of several patients whom we interviewed. This is the discrepancy between the statement that one minimum dose will be sufficient for a cure and the fact that most of our interviewees have been given several treatments over an extended period of time. The consumer must be prepared for extended treatment if the condition calls for it. Even though this may be disappointing to some, it is actually safer than the "miracle cure" impression one garners from the promotional literature. Most of those we have interviewed have completely recovered and have not experienced a recurrence of the same condition.

Sources to Read

Periodicals

Homeopathy
PO Box 3100
San Francisco, CA 94131

Homoeopathic Heartbeat
7297-H Lee Highway
Falls Church, VA 22042

The Homeopathic Digest
PO Box 667
Ossining, NY 10562

Journal of the American Institute of Homeopathy
6231 Leesburg Pike, Suite 506
Falls Church, VA 22044

Books

Baker, Wryth P., M.D., M.H.D., F.A.C.D., D-HT. *Fundamentals of Homoeotherapeutics, Part I and II.* Falls Church, VA: National Center for Homoeopathy, 1977.

Clarke, John Henry. *Prescriber.* Rustington, Sussex, England: Health Science Press, 1972.

Coulter, Harris, Ph.D. *The Divided Legacy.* Washington, DC: Wehawken Books, 1973.

———. *Homoeopathic Medicine.* St. Louis, MO: Formur, 1973.

Gibson, D. M. *First Aid Homeopathy in Accidents and Ailments.* London, England: British Homeopathic Association, 1975.

Gutman, William, M.D. *Homeopathy, The Fundamentals of Its Philosophy: The Essence of Its Remedies.* Santa Cruz, CA: The Homoeopathy Medical Publishers, 1978.

Hahnemann, Samuel. *Organon of Medicine.* Boulder, CO: Hermes Press, 1977.

Hall, Manly Palmer. *Mystical and Medical Philosophy of Paracelsus.* Los Angeles, CA: Philosophical Research Society, 1964.

Kaufman, Martin. *Homeopathy in America: The Rise and Fall of a Medical Heresy.* Baltimore, MD: Johns Hopkins Press, 1971.

Millspaugh, Charles F., M.D. *American Medicinal Plants.* New York: Dover, 1974.

Mitchell, George Rughven. *Homeopathy: The First Authoritative Study of Its Place in Medicine Today.* London: W. H. Allen, 1975.

National Center for Homoeopathy. *Expand Your Knowledge of Homoeotherapeutics.* Falls Church, VA: National Center for Homoeopathy, n.d.

Panos, Maesimund, M.D., and **Heimlich, J.** *Homeopathic Medicine at Home: Natural Remedies for Everyday Ailments and Minor Injuries.* New York: J. P. Tarcher, 1980.

Selye, Hans. "Self Regulation: The Response to Stress," *Inner Balance.* ed. E. M. Goldwag, Englewood Cliffs, NJ: Prentice-Hall, 1979.

———. *The Stress of Life.* New York: McGraw-Hill Book Company, 1976.

Shadman, Alonzo J. *Who Is Your Doctor and Why?* St. Louis: Former International, 1958.

Sharma, Gandra H. *A Manual of Homeopathy and Natural Medicine.* New York: Dutton, 1975.

Shepherd, Dorothy. *Magic of Minimum Dose.* Rustington, Sussex, England: Health Science Press, 1964.

——. *More Magic of Minimum Dose.* Rustington, Sussex, England: Health Science Press, 1969.

Simonton, Carl O., Matthews-Simonton, S., and **Creighton, C.** *Getting Well Again.* Los Angeles: J. P. Tarcher, Inc., 1978.

Vargo, Kay. "What is Homoeopathy?" Falls Church, VA: National Center for Homoeopathy, 1975.

Vithoulkas, George. "Homeopathy" in *The Holistic Health Handbook*, ed. Edward Brint et al. Berkeley, CA: And/Or Press, 1978.

——. *Homeopathy, Medicine of the New Man: A Complete Introduction to the Natural System of Medicine.* New York: Avon Books, 1972.

Voegeli, Adolph. *Homeopathic Prescribing.* Northants, England: Thorsons, 1976.

5

ACUPUNCTURE

Definition

Acupuncture is the science of balancing bodily energies still practiced by women medics, barefoot doctors, and M.D.'s in China. Its methods are based upon ancient Taoist philosophy and were used at least two thousand years before the birth of Christ. In the strictest sense it has been trusted as long as any healing method known to man. To the ancient Chinese all contents of the universe and all phenomena contained the life force, an energy considered the basis of life. This "vital energy" is similar to some of the other conceptions of the "vital force" found among such holistic healers examined in this book as naturopaths and homoeopaths. The major difference between the theory underlying acupuncture and those that form the basis for these other modalities is that the ancient Chinese elaborated upon their concept during their long history of experimentation with it.

  Yin and *yang* are the dual components of *Chi* (the life energy). They are as opposite as night and day and are symbolically represented within all entities. These interconnected forces are capable of creating either balance or imbalance in the vital energy (Chi) of the body.

Yin and yang are analogous to the mathematical concepts of positive and negative as well as the electrical impulses of + and −. When both energies are operating, they cancel each other out and equal 0. Zero is the perfect balance of yin and yang in the life force. An excess or a deficiency in either energy creates dis-ease in the body (Acupuncture Research Institute, 1975; Chen, 1969; Lavier, 1974; Lawson-Wood, 1973; Manaka and Urquhard, 1972).

Traditionally, yin has symbolized the feminine characteristics of receptiveness, passivity, and secretiveness, whereas yang has represented the masculine characteristics of aggressiveness, activeness, and openness. The beginning of dis-ease is yang, symbolizing symptoms that show themselves externally. Dis-ease that locates itself within the body is considered yin. When dis-ease occurs, the characteristics appear in terms that describe the imbalance and locate its manifestations in the body.

The "Chi," or "life force," is carried in the physical body through what acupuncturists call *meridians*. Practitioners explain that meridians map a geography of the body and run from head to toe and side to side. In a manner of speaking, the life force travels down highways of meridians. Loci are points located below the surface of the skin along the meridians. Acupuncturists detect the proper point and stabilize the imbalance in the yin and yang by relaxing or stimulating specific loci for specific symptoms. It might be said that the healer can reach the Chi by way of loci. A loci is equivalent to a train station along a meridian highway. The Chi (life energy) travels through meridians and is contacted and balanced through loci along its path.

When applying the philosophy of acupuncture to practical treatment methods, it is more comprehensive than just yin, yang, and Chi. This definition of the underlying symbols of the system of healing, therefore, is only a thumbnail sketch. More complex aspects of the philosophy begin when considering a few of the dis-ease processes associated with these concepts.

The Chinese observed that Chi flowed in two major cycles, generative and destructive. Furthermore, they saw that the generative and destructive cycles of energy mirrored five elements of earth: fire, earth, metal, water, and wood. This means that each element creates or destroys the action of the one following it. Elements are associated with specific organs, bowels, or the heart. Interrelated organs and bowels are linked along the paths of meridians, thereby allowing interdependence as treatment of one affects treatment of another. For example, attending the small intestine, which is associated with fire, automatically leads to relief in the stomach (earth). The process is a chain reaction that affects bowels and organs in its path. (Chang, 1976)

Since acupuncture is philosophical, practical, and complicated, the making of an acupuncturist is a long and tedious process. Holistic practitioners report that they must be proficient in herbs, acupressure, exercise, moxibustion, massage, heat therapy, and nutrition and how they interrelate, in addition to understanding and applying these basic components to processes of dis-ease. In China even potential allopathic physicians learn acupuncture. Each must become cognizant of the mapping of meridians and loci and the interworkings of the earthly elements.

We found that acupuncturists distinguish themselves as either "traditional" or "modern" based upon their training in methods of diagnosis and treatment. Until 1955 they were trained in traditional or natural ways. Technology affected the training and, consequently, the practices of those professionals trained after 1955. Electrical vibrators, extreme variations in needle size, and automatic point locators are but a few of the mechanical devices offered to acupuncturists by modern technology. Many (both traditional and modern) believe that these techniques may appear to be sophisticated, necessary to progress, or even used to impress the patient as to the "validity" of acupuncture and/or the practitioner. Along with these "gadgets" emerged the belief that drugs may be necessary in order to treat dis-ease.

There are major belief differences between orthodox Western physicians and orthodox Eastern acupuncturists concerning the ways in which dis-ease is viewed. Even though most physicians admit awareness of "a larger force" within the patient and are learned in the functioning of homeostasis, as far as we know, few conventional practitioners acknowledge the presence of Chi or yin or yang. Acupuncturists believe that Chi is a spiritual life force that is the basis of health with yin and yang characteristics. Western physicians, according to Oriental healers, treat only physical symptoms, thereby denying the spiritual aspects of the disease. Therefore, if physicians do not believe in life force as asserted by acupuncturists, they do not believe that yin and yang features play an important role in determining how dis-ease is remedied. Furthermore, acupuncturists point out that loci and meridians are viewed by doctors as nonexistent, and hypnosis and suggestion are seen as the primary reason for acupuncture's success, even in light of research that validates previous "word of mouth" accounts. But the most belittling comment about acupuncture made by the medical community is that it is "the profession where malpractice insurance wouldn't do any good." The bias resides in both acupuncture and organized medicine and is something a consumer must expect within this holistic practice.

While studying the field of acupuncture, we came across a start-
ling amount of evidence that supported its curative powers. Although
preliminary data from Western research projects have been reported in
the U.S., most scientific statistical information has been published elsewhere. The body of evidence long ago exposed the fact that acupuncture
proved extremely valuable in treating many different varieties of
dis-ease.

In 1959 250 patients in the Soviet Union, with eleven different
illnesses, who are purported to have been unsuccessfully treated by
Western doctors, were cured or greatly improved following acupuncture
therapy. Another Soviet physician cured or improved 195 people who
were also purported to have been unsuccessfully treated by Western
physicians. In 1960 three Russian physicians reported that 26 out of 35
were cured, and follow-up studies revealed that the cures continued in
all but 3 of the patients. A French physician treated over a five-year
period 625 patients who had been unsuccessfully treated by Western
doctors. It was reported that 525 of his patients were cured of 108
different illnesses. According to all the researchers, no drugs were used
in these experiments, only needles (Duke, 1973).

Acupuncturists report that successful experimentation is often
neglected due to the presupposition that acupuncture is a form of
hypnosis or suggestion (see Austin, 1975; Chen, 1969; Croizer, 1968;
Huard and Wong, 1968). Dr. Thomas Mann, a British physician, tried to
prove that psychology did not affect acupuncture's rate of cure by
drugging his patients before applying treatment so that hypnosis or
suggestion could not account for the success. He successfully treated
over 1,200 diseases (Duke, 1973).

One of the major triumphs of acupuncture is its treatment of Type
B encephalitis. As stated by Marc Duke:

> Using only acupuncture, Chinese physicians treat Type B encephalitis, a
> disease the West can do little to cure. When it strikes, Type B encephalitis
> often causes paralysis. Sometimes it kills. By 1953 Chinese acupuncturists
> had achieved a 95% cure rate of patients who caught it. The treatment is
> not available to Americans who contract Type B encephalitis. Most U.S.
> physicians are unaware that an effective cure for the disease exists. Since
> they rely upon A.M.A. Journal's information, and it has chosen to remain
> silent, their ignorance is understandable—although for people with Type
> B encephalitis, far from acceptable [Duke, 1973].

Finally, as early as 1963, a Korean doctor discovered variations in skin
resistance and cell structure on points traced along meridians that were
drawn long ago by Chinese practitioners (Chang, 1976). Before and since
that time, other research has only been able to confirm that temperature
differs and that skin is less dense at acupuncture points (Duke, 1973;

Warren, 1976). Loci, then, do not contain the same characteristics as the rest of the skin and their existence has been verified empirically, unless we are to think that these experiments were deliberately falsified.

However, because of the lack of evidence being produced here and because of an increasing number of unreliable acupuncturists in the Western market, medical organizations have felt the need to establish guidelines for acupuncture practitioners in the U.S. Many precautions are now taken by governmental and professional medical organizations. The FDA and the healing arts licensing boards called a meeting on September 22, 1972, in Washington. Representatives from the American Medical Association, American Society of Anesthesiologists, Federation of State Medical Boards, the National Institutes of Health, and selected "interested parties" attended. They decided by the "unanimous consensus of those attending the meeting that the use of acupuncture constitutes an experimental procedure and the equipment used—needles and electrical generators for stimulation—are experimental devices" (Warren, 1976).

Because Western practitioners have so little experience with acupuncture, the medical establishment and state governments have taken a skeptical view of the field. Acupuncture is, indeed, a complex science that speaks and treats in terms uncommon to us. It was developed by observation and grounded in a philosophy that centers on interrelationships between people, society, nature, the universe, and health. Acupuncture is difficult simply because our culture does not exemplify these elements. To the Chinese it is quite natural to base healing upon the life force. As you read this book, notice that it is given many different names but encompasses the same definition.

Type of Healing

Originally, acupuncture was a natural healing method. By *natural* we mean that healers were trained in the traditional philosophy of acupuncture, practiced those methods, and had little use for most modern scientific medicines. Much of it is still natural, but, as we have mentioned, this depends upon the professional you choose, the beliefs he or she holds about acupuncture, and the manner in which a specific healer has been trained. The distinction between natural (traditional) and technological (modern) acupuncture may make your decision to use it difficult.

There are frequent crossovers within the profession. Traditional acupuncturists proclaim advantages of some advances made by technology and do make use of these products. Modern acupuncturists have also made a "step backward" in that they are more likely to use herbs, exercise, and counseling. By and large, practitioners are combining the "best" methods of the past with the "best" methods of the present.

Acupuncture is most commonly associated with needles. No one has explained the reasons why it was felt that needles were so essential to healing. But healers are taught many different methods to heal. Among these and as important as needle treatment, but one which is rarely mentioned, is herbal therapy. Nearly all acupuncturists treat imbalances with herbal remedies. Some potions can contain one or two herbs. Practitioners explain these are not prepackaged medicine but are mixed for each individual so as to balance the vital energies specifically.

Acupuncture method, as well as the devices and needles used for treatment, are labeled "experimental" by the experts. Some individual state governments are given the power to restrict professional practices, most states require that acupuncturists be licensed. Other states allow acupuncturists to practice either in hospitals or clinics under the supervision of licensed M.D.'s. These constrictions are to protect reliable practitioners as well as unknowing consumers from charlatans.

Potential healers study herbal medicine alongside acupuncture diagnosis and treatment methods. Acupuncturists explain that the alkaline-producing effects of herbs can prevent many illnesses. Additionally, healers point out that herbs are mixed according to the yin or yang characteristics and are comparable with the Western ways of prescription. For example, the basic herb with curative effects is called the *emperir*. Its aid is called the *ministor*. The catalyst plant that helps carry the whole remedy is called the *ambassador* (Duke, 1973). Although given different names, prescribed mixtures are composed in the same manner within structured medicine.

Another important part of acupuncture is pulse diagnosis. According to traditional acupuncturists, the pulse method takes years of training before it can be understood. This method enables practitioners to diagnose past dis-eases as well as present and future energy imbalances within a body. There are six pulses on each wrist, twelve pulses in all. Depending upon whether the pulse is felt on the top, in the middle, or on the bottom, pulses lead the practitioner to one or more of twelve organs that may show energy imbalances. Practitioners who make use of these pulses for diagnosis express that subtleties in the rate of pulse are very hard to detect but that the life force communicates through them. This method of diagnosis is under extreme criticism from modern practitioners as one of the least practical and most ridiculous methods practiced. However, traditional acupuncturists violently disagree. They feel that it is the most encompassing of all the methods.

Description of Healing Method

Thus far we have avoided discussing the use of *needles* in acupuncture because of the stigma associated with them. We know that knowledge of the subject should be the basis upon which one chooses acupuncture rather than feelings regarding the use of needles. As you can tell from our discussion, there is a complex philosophy underlying the therapy of needles. Perhaps this is presumptuous on our part, but unless one is an advocate of pain, needles are to be avoided at any cost.

In addition to herbs and massage, the use of needles is the major method of acupuncturists. Needles can be utilized in many ways. They are stainless steel and range in size from one to eight inches. As it was explained to us, the initial "stick" is called "getting the spirit" (Chi). In this way the practitioner is grabbing the attention of the spirit. Once the attention is gained, acupuncturists must communicate with the spirit by way of the needle. The needle maneuvers the yin and yang, which in turn maneuver the body's healing abilities while the mind is aware of the whole process. Spirit, mind, and body are thereby stimulated both consciously and unconsciously.

We were careful to find out how the needle procedure felt to the healee. Many healees that we interviewed report that no pain is felt after the first needle is inserted. Others report that, in the case of electrical acupuncture, one is aware of the needle for as long as 20 minutes before numbing occurs. Overall, healees point out that only a slight discomfort is felt. We have summarized from our questioning what to expect below so that consumers may judge for themselves.

A Needling Feeling

When the needle is first inserted, you will experience a slight "ouch" reaction. You should then experience a tingling feeling around that area. The tingling feeling will then change into heaviness. You may notice some swelling, but not all people do. The area around the needle will turn red, and, at this time, you should notice a warm feeling around the needle. When the needle is manipulated, the warm feeling is extended to numbness. The numbness is spread to the infected part or through the whole body. Pain should be nonexistent after the first needle which has entered an acupuncture point, when analgesia, freeing the body from pain, is produced.

Some other techniques used with acupuncture needles are as follows:

tonification—stimulation of the body's vital forces
sedation—a decrease of the body's life forces

twirled needle—needles are twirled to produce increased numbness or pain relief

vibrated needles—can be done with a vibrator or electricity to increase the effects and produce longer-lasting results

dextro rotations—turning to the right—and laevo rotations—turning to the left; these two are used for setting up opposing electrical fields in the body.

Holistic acupuncturists claim that needles are not the "mainstay" of acupuncture, for whole-person treatment does not rely upon one single method. When an acupuncture practitioner examines you, he or she is assessing interrelationships of the natural balance of spirit, mind, body, emotions, and environment. The first visit with these practitioners is lengthy because of the time alloted for diagnosis of dis-ease.

Be prepared for a feeling of being scrutinized at first. So-called "standard" identifications are made through the family's medical history, personal medical history, definitions, and descriptions of the complaint. But, many other areas are also studied in an acupuncture examination. An acupuncturist is trained as an acute observer. He or she is aware of your breathing, voice, posture, diet, hair, skin, excretions, and even the colors of your body. Previous clients report that your feelings and dreams are questioned for insight into yin-yang traits of the dis-ease as well as symbols assigned to the dis-ease by the healee.

In many cases, *acupressure* is used in place of needles. This may serve to mitigate many of your fears. According to healers, relief through practice of acupressure can be felt by placing fingertip pressure on the correct loci. This asserted pressure produces an effect similar to needles. One of the advantages of acupressure is that it is easily learned and can be used to maintain the balance of Chi. Interestingly, acupressure has been integrated into other natural methods, such as massage and chiropractic.

Moxibustion is still another method used widely by acupuncture practitioners. Moxibustion consists of using the dried seed or leaves of the mugwort plant. The seed is placed on the end of the injected needle and lit. The heat travels through the needle and into the body. The mugwort seed, healers point out, is employed to relieve spasms, cramps, and swellings and to increase urine. Other practitioners place the leaves on the correct point, light them, and remove them before a burn appears. A burn can leave a scar, which will affect the flow of the vital force. Before using this method, practitioners first test to see if the skin is sensitive. If it is any consolation, acupuncturists are taught to practice this method on themselves so that it will be perfected before he or she tries it on someone else. You should only feel a "sting." It is used to supplement or tone a yang dis-ease. The curative effects of the burning herb have not yet been explored by science.

Heat and massage are also used regularly as treatment. Sauna, hot towels, and hot poultices offer methods that are easily assimilated into preventive life-style practices. Massage gives relaxation and stimulation simultaneously. During a massage, a practitioner can use fingers, knuckles, toes, and heels of the hand to produce the desired effects. Acupuncturists express that these simple methods can have the largest "payoff" when taking a step toward maintaining health.

Remember that changes in dietary habits and exercise facilitate acupuncture. Furthermore, holistic acupuncturists will teach deep-breathing exercises and meditation as well as acupressure to the healee so that exchange between spirit, mind, and body manifests itself in a natural manner. Therefore, the preventive nature of acupuncture is consistent with holistic practices because its techniques are easily added to the home environment.

Most acupuncture clinics ask that a consumer sign a contract. This contract entitles you to any information regarding your care. It protects both patient and practitioner by clearly defining the roles and responsibilities of medical treatment. Your contract will state a common purpose and describe what is necessary to fulfill the plan. In this way you actively participate in the healing program as well as its outcome.

To restore your body to health entails a comprehensive program. Previous clients affirm that practitioners teach you how to manage the yin and yang—that is, your health. Additionally, healees told us that they were asked to exercise daily so that their muscles do not become flabby from inactivity. Like chiropractic practitioners and massage therapists, acupuncturists are of the belief that exercise and good posture are vitally important in preventing future dis-ease. One set of exercises called the Five Animals Game was reported by a healee as an example of implementation of exercise into acupuncture. In the first part of the exercise your body is still and breathing. This is practiced until breath is steady and slow. The second part of the game consists of imitating a bear, a stag, a monkey, a tiger, and a crane according to your visual perception of the animal's activity. According to this former client, these help ensure a long and healthy life and balance the yin and yang.

Your diet is surveyed carefully for incorrect mixtures of foods that may produce an energy imbalance. Most practitioners ask that you list the foods you eat on a regular basis as well as those you snack on and those that you drink. Acupuncturists recommend that weight be kept within seven pounds of what it was when you were twenty-five years old. This, it is suggested, can be accomplished by a few simple rules. Eat only what is needed and do not overeat. Chew your food well. Avoid salt, white sugar, white flour. Eat plenty of fresh fruits and vegetables and eat only lean meats.

By the time a diagnosis is made, the practitioner has located the troubled yin or yang area. Treatment follows immediately and you are not rescheduled for treatment on another day. Cure is described by acupuncturists as immediate. In many cases acupuncturists point out, future visitations are not often necessary. Exercise, diet, acupressure, and massage are preventive measures that enhance acupuncture treatment and help maintain balance. Living simple is acupuncture's rule to follow. Holistic practitioners in this field express that life should be joyful, not viewed as a hassle. To them happiness is a fundamental building block of a healthy life-style. Both healers and healees assert that attitude and personal habits, you see, are as powerful preventions of dis-ease as needles are powerful cures.

Diseases Treated

Most of the dis-eases treated by acupuncturists are nerve blockages. However, the list of illnesses is extensive: dental pain, facial pain, arthritis, nerve injuries, chronic and acute pain, surgical recovery, eyestrain, headaches, prostrate conjection, torticolis, cervical herpes, causalgia, acute vascular occlusion, cerebral accidents, herpes zoster, TBC laryngitis, limitation of shoulder and arm, angina, frostbite, hyperhydrosis, bronchial asthma, paroxysmal tachycardia, fractured ribs, idiopathy chest pains, fractures of costal cartilage, thrombophlebitis, artherial occlusion, Hirschsprung's disease, chronic ulcers, sciatica, lower back pain, blood pressure, minor fractures, postoperative scars, phlebothrombosis, chronic peripheral vascular disease, salpingitis, coccygodynia, gangrene, lumbago, gout, tennis elbow, hay fever, renal colic, tinnitus, tracheitis, Parkinson's disease, eczema, seborrhea, anemia, rheumatism, migraines, sinusitis, neuralgia, circulation, anxiety, fear, pleurisy, parotitis, spasms, toothache, depression, diarrhea, obesity, vertigo, apoplexy, boils, bronchitis, chills, cold, constipation, nephritis, nosebleeds, pyorrhea, colitis, cystitis, involuntary erection, fatigue, pneumonia, emphysema, gastritis, hernia, insomnia, vaginitis, hypertension, psoriasis, blurred vision, dizziness.

Acupuncture is especially effective for the treatment of pain, headaches, arthritis, postoperative pain, acute pain, and chronic pain. It has been used successfully for high blood pressure, chronic ulcers, and dental pain, but its effectiveness may be due to a combination of treatments. Practitioners have had little success with cancer, tuberculosis, or degenerative nerve diseases.

Duration of Treatment

Previous healees reported dental pain, headaches, arthritis, and post-operative pain are easily relieved immediately. Most clients do not feel the need to return to an acupuncturist for further treatment. However, many acupuncturists declare that whereas cures of chronic and acute suffering take longer and pain can be removed immediately, more visits are needed to erect a preventive wall against recurrence. Minor problems, according to healers, usually take one or two visits, whereas more serious problems can take between eight and twenty visits. Of course, your energy balance must be maintained, which means that compliance with the recommendations given by the healer will have to be carried out.

If you have been referred to an acupuncturist by a physician, your treatment will be exactly what is recommended and nothing else. Unless you specifically point out that you do not feel that your diagnosis is based on spirit, mind, and body, the practitioner will not necessarily involve you in much "detail" for the treatment. Practitioners of acupuncture do not want to "overstep" their boundaries in conventional medical fields. Therefore, you must listen carefully for "hints" given about your dis-ease and question ideas that you feel may be related to your problem.

Healees describe first visits as lengthy because of the detailed information required before treatment is given. This questioning process takes approximately two hours and includes a physical examination. Treatments take about thirty minutes. Of course this can vary. Massage, acupressure, and heat treatments may take somewhat longer. If your acupuncturist is competent, you will not have to keep returning for treatments because you will be able to distinguish imbalances and rectify them. It takes an average of three trips to a practitioner to learn the procedures one is to follow at home. Interestingly enough, some healers charge clients for preventive instruction and others do not.

Cost Range

There are many acupuncturists that charge exorbitant fees. It is interesting to note that fees have increased since 1965. This appears to be due to increased demand, increased technology in the field and increased numbers of Western physicians in the field. If one is located in California, New York, or Washington, D.C., you will find the prices lower because of the number of professionals and professional clinics located in these areas. We feel that it is better to go to a clinic that employs acupuncturists because these fees are a set price, regardless of the treatment. This is because there are a number of practitioners available in the holistic field and because there is a cooperative "preventive" attitude among them. Therefore, we have compared prices of acupuncture clinics with those of individual physicians.

	CLINIC	INDIVIDUAL
Initial visit:	$30–$40	donation–$45
Follow-up visit:	$30–$40	donation–$35
Acupuncture (straight):	$30–$40	donation–$100
Electrical acupuncture:	$30–$40	donation–$100
Acupressure:	$30–$40	donation–$30
Twirled needles:	$30–$40	donation–$50
Massage:	$30–$35	donation–$35
Sedation, tonification, etc.:	$30–$40	donation–$100
Counseling:	included free	included free
Heat massage:	$30–$40	donation–$45
Moxa (moxibustion):	$30–$45	donation–$55
Meridian massage:	$30–$40	donation–$35

Personal Responsibilities

As with other holistic methods, much of the healing in acupuncture is your responsibility. However, you are somewhat less responsible in acupuncture than in other methods simply because practitioners are taught that a good acupuncturist *prevents dis-ease before it occurs*. But, you won't get off that easy. You are responsible for planning a holistic acupuncture program that includes mental health, diet, exercise, maintenance of energy balance, and self-examination. Furthermore, these facets of health are to be implemented into your life-style to promote health and well-being.

Because of the "experimental" nature of acupuncture, it is best to protect your and the practitioner's interests by signing an informed consent. Some practitioners do not use them, and therefore, they should be avoided. The form should explain your treatment in detail, in terms that are understandable to you, as well as of any dangerous side effects that might possibly result from treatment. Holistic acupuncturists often require the healee to record his or her own responsibilities for the cure in addition to the description and dangers of acupuncture. Informed consents might be required in all holistic fields in order to ensure consumer awareness about the method. Please be aware that an informed consent *does not* have any legal benefits for the healee or for the practitioner. Do not forget to check if acupuncturists must be licensed in your state.

If you are being treated for a prolonged period of time, you should become proficient in diagnosing life forces. This preventive procedure is usually taught by holistic practitioners and provides clues to imbalances in yin and yang. If imbalances are discovered ahead of time, one can easily avoid dis-ease by self-correcting or a trip to the healer. A small amount of time will have to be spent each day in order to rebalance your vital force. Several techniques, such as exercise, massage, heat, and acupressure, are taught to help you accomplish this aspect of acupuncture. It is crucial that you accept the responsibility for self-care measures furnished by the acupuncturist. As in any holistic health method, without your taking active steps in the direction of health, a holistic practitioner cannot further your personal quest for ease.

Appropriate life-styles—that is, life-styles that promote good health—will also be your responsibility. Acupuncturists support the belief that simple living is healthier than the hectic life most of us lead in today's complex world. This concept is complicated in that simple living has many connotations. But the bottom line, so to speak, indicates that simple living means less emotional involvement in problems, a less competitive life-style, less concern for time, better dietary habits, fulfillment of personal purposes, and a certain joy about life.

Informational Organizations

It is nearly impossible to find out about acupuncture from their professional organizations. After many unanswered letters and phone messages left with answering services, we still did not receive any information from them. We can only suggest that you try a state organization or writing for information from one of the centers in the following list. The clinic setting is much more helpful to consumers.

Center for Traditional Acupuncture, Inc.
The American City Building
Columbia, MD 21044

Center for Chinese Medicine
PO Box 32072
Los Angeles, CA 90032

National Acupuncture Association
PO Box 24509
Los Angeles, CA 90024

Consistencies

1. Traditional acupuncturists are what sociologists call folk healers. That is, their medicine is medicine of the people—a set of beliefs and behaviors practiced by everyone. Ancient Chinese (Taoist) beliefs emphasized treatment of the spirit, mind, body, and emotions in a natural manner. This method is therefore consistent with the holistic philosophy.

2. Unlike most folk healers, the acupuncturist receives a diploma after years of apprenticeship under a Chinese physician. This training process is designed to assure quality among traditional practitioners.

3. The diagnostic procedures used by acupuncturists allow for a more thorough understanding of dis-ease. As we mentioned in the preceding text, the depth of their diagnosis extends throughout all spheres of a person's life and includes several methods, not a single procedure.

4. Many miracle "cures" have been attributed to acupuncture. We have discussed how Type B encephalitis, considered incurable by Western physicians, has an extremely high cure rate among acupuncturists. Perhaps the extensive holistic nature of Chinese philosophy and its long history are two reasons why miracles are possible. After all, it is the longest known medical experiment in the history of humankind.

5. Many practitioners will accept a donation as a fee. This serves to alleviate the high cost of acupuncture.

6. Diet, exercise, and life-style changes are designed and implemented by the client in cooperation with the healer. This program of total care allows one to individualize the health program. Equal responsibility between consumers and healers is also consistent with holism.

7. Acupuncturists maintain that you are responsible for the balance and imbalance of the vital force in your own life. You are taught preventive measures, self-diagnosis, and techniques for restoration or balance of vital energies.

8. Throughout holistic practices, healers employ the use of the informed consent form. Acupuncture is no exception. A health contract can also accompany this document to spell out the details of consumer/healer responsibilities.

Inconsistencies

1. Some modern acupuncturists tend to disregard in practice the philosophy of the whole. These are primarily physicians who are new to the acupuncture healing system and who use the acupuncture procedure because it works. Because of their training and beliefs, most do not practice the more traditional philosophy and are more concerned with establishing the legitimacy of the treatment within the confines of conventional medical practice.

2. It is unlikely that most Westerners seeking Chinese medicine would find a Chinese physician. "Outsiders" are viewed with suspicion and are barred from most Chinese institutions. This even extends to professional organizations. They do not support the consumer by answering mail or returning phone calls. Cultural barriers between the more traditional Chinese and the rest of the consumer public will have to be overcome before this inconsistency can be resolved.

3. Most of the medical profession has "blackballed" acupuncturists in spite of research that supports its curative powers. Some doctors who have made use of acupuncture in the past have lost their jobs. Doctors that practice it can lose their jobs. Whatever the specific reason for the Western bias against such holistic treatments as acupuncture, consumers are the ones who lose.

4. There are few training procedures available to Western physicians who may wish to try and learn about it. This only reinforces the Chinese belief that we are "outsiders" and prevents the assimilation of Eastern and Western medicine.

5. Practitioners are not adequately distributed throughout the United States. They usually practice in large cities where there is a Chinese community. This limits the availability of their services.

6. All of this adds up to a situation where the layman is denied access to knowledge about acupuncture. The best way for you to learn about this method is to read books on the subject or to question practitioners themselves. We suggest, however, that you avoid using any needles until you visit a licensed practitioner and receive adequate guidance.

7. With current ongoing research projects in the U.S., orthodox physicians are becoming aware of acupuncture's curative abilities. Physicians, for the most part, realize that their therapies must be expanded in order to treat the wide range of dis-eases experienced by consumers. Unfortunately the bias held by acupuncturists against physicians and vice versa circumvents scientific findings.

Sources to Read

Academy of Traditional Chinese Medicine. *An Outline of Chinese Acupuncture.* San Francisco: China Books, 1975.

Acupuncture Research Institute. *Acupuncture Made Easy.* Alhambra, CA: Chan's Books, 1975.

Austin, Mary. *Acupuncture Therapy.* New York: ASI, 1975.

Cerney, J. V. *Acupressure: Acupuncture without Needles.* Englewood Cliffs, NJ: Prentice-Hall, 1973.

Chan, Pedro. *Electro-Acupuncture: Its Clinical Application in Therapy.* Alhambra, CA: Chan's Books, 1974.

———. *Finger Acupressure.* Alhambra, CA: Chan's Books, 1975.

———. *Wonders of Chinese Acupuncture.* Alhambra, CA: Borden, 1973.

Chang, Stephen. *Complete Book of Acupuncture.* Millbrae, CA: Celestial Arts, 1976.

Chen, Ronald. *The History and Methods of Physical Diagnosis in Classical Chinese Medicine.* New York: Vantage, 1969.

Croizier, Ralph C. *Traditional Medicine in Modern China.* Cambridge, Mass: Howard D. Press, 1968.

Dornette, William H. L. "Acupuncture and the Law," *Journal of Legal Medicine* 2, no. 2 (March–April 1974): 31–38.

Duke, Marc. *Acupuncture.* New York: Pyramid, 1973.

Greene, Foly. *Awakened China.* Garden City, NY: Doubleday, 1961.

Hellerman, Leon, and **Stein, Alan L.**, eds. *China: Readings on the Middle Kingdom.* New York: Simon and Schuster, 1971.

Houston, F. M. *Healing Benefits of Acupressure.* New Caanan, CT: Keats, 1974.

Huang-ti Nei Chung Su Wen. *The Yellow Emperor's Classic of Internal Medicine*, trans. Iza Veith. Berkeley, CA: University of California Press, 1966; reprinted 1972.

Huard, Pierre, and **Wong, Ming.** *Chinese Medicine*, trans. Bernard Fielding. New York: McGraw-Hill, 1968.

Hwang, Paul T. K.; Wong, Joshua S. L.; and **Chan, Pedro C. P.** *Acupuncture Made Easy.* Alhambra, CA: Chan's Books, 1975.

Langre, Jacques de. *First Book of Do-In.* Wethersfield, CT: Omangod, 1973.

Lavier, J. *Points of Chinese Acupuncture*, trans. Phillip M. Chancellor. Wellingborough, England: Health Science Press, 1974.

Lawson-Wood, Denis. *Acupuncture and Chinese Massage.* Rustington, England: Health Services Press, 1965.

———. *Acupuncture Handbook.* New York: Weiser, 1973.

Man, Pang L. *Handbook of Acupuncture Analgesia.* Woodbury, NJ: Field Place Press, 1973.

Manaka, Yoshio, and **Urquhard, Ian A.** *The Layman's Guide to Acupuncture.* New York: Weatherhill, 1972.

Mann, Felix. *Acupuncture: The Ancient Chinese Art of Healing.* Westminister, MD: Random House, 1974.

———. *Acupuncture: Cure of Many Diseases.* Boston: Tao Books, 1972.

———. *The Treatment of Disease by Acupuncture and Body Energies.* Phoenix, AZ: Gabriel Press, 1974.

Moss, Louis. *Acupuncture and You.* London: Elek Books, 1964.

Needham, Joseph, and **Kuei-jen, Lu.** "Hygiene and Preventive Medicine in Ancient China," *Journal of the History of Medicine and Allied Sciences* 18 (October 1962): 429–78.

Palos, Stephan. *The Chinese Art of Healing.* New York: Bantam, 1972.

Stiefvater, Erick N. *What Is Acupuncture: How Does It Work?* Rushington, Sussex, England: Health Science Press, 1962.

Tan, Leong T.; Margaret, Y. C., and **Veith, Ilza.** *Acupuncture Therapy, Current Chinese Practice*, 2d ed. Philadelphia: Temple University Press, 1976.

U.S., Department of Health, Education and Welfare. *A Barefoot Doctors Manual.* Washington, D.C.: DHEW Publications (NIH) 75-695 (1974).

Wallnofer, Heinrich, and **Rottauscher, Anna von.** *Chinese Folk Medicine.* New York: Bell Publishing Co., 1965.

Warren, Frank Z. *Handbook of Medical Acupuncture.* New York: Van Nostrand Reinhold, 1976.

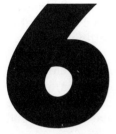

CHIROPRACTIC

Definition

Holistic chiropractors maintain that the body, like nature, is self-regulating and that healing is brought about by the body as long as it is functionally and structurally balanced. This balance is important because chiropractors feel that the relationship between the spine and the nervous system is a key factor in keeping the curative channels of the body open. Chiropractors believe that dis-eases can be caused by disturbances in the nervous system, which can be upset by derangements of the musculoskeletal structure. This, in turn, may cause problems in other systems in the body.

They also believe that the mind plays an important role in any healing process because it is within the healee that motivation and ability for health begin. Since the power of maintaining health is contained within each of us, our own attitudes and life-styles are important factors. Responsibility for health is placed upon the healee, and responsibility for motivating the patient is accepted by the healer. In this context the most challenging patient is an apathetic one.

The chiropractic profession has been criticized by the medical profession for years. However, claims that chiropractic is "dangerous" and "does more harm than good" appear to be unfounded. Otherwise, the sheer number of consumers who are satisfied with this field are wrong. One reason for the satisfaction may, in fact, be what one holistic chiropractor told us: "We teach a preventive life-style and demand that patients stop taking medication and change their attitudes toward disease."

According to the American Chiropractic Association, chiropractors have rigorous scientific standards that must be met. In order to maintain these standards, most state chiropractic associations require continued education for licensing. All fifty states have approved and licensed chiropractors.

Pardon the pun, but according to chiropractors, your spine is the "backbone" of health. As explained to us, the spinal column contains twenty-four movable vertebrae, elastic cartilage plates (spinal disks), and ligaments with muscles around it. Nerves run the entire length of the spine throughout all these parts. Normally, the spine with all of its related segments, moves freely. When movement is erratic, these free-moving divisions often get "stuck" or "locked," causing not only an odd posture but also pain and irritation in the nervous system. Chiropractors point out that *subluxation* or a *fixation* is a mechanical lesion in the nervous system at the point where nerves exit or enter the spinal column. A subluxation, simply put, is a partly displaced vertebrae, and a fixation is a partly restricted vertebrae. Either one of these contribute to disorders that affect both "structural balance" and "functional tone." R. C. Shafer, D.C. says that the corrective adjustment necessary to correct this disorder is a surface technique that is "light-touch reflex adjustments . . . much akin . . . to Chinese meridian therapy," which is rarely if ever painful. Dr. Schafer maintains that a disturbance in the spine needs to be dealt with from a holistic perspective because it might lead to disorders in other areas of the body or the body as a whole (1977).

Dintenfass (1970) describes the experience of a subluxation by the client as a feeling of a "crick" or a "click" in the back due to abnormal movements or injury. These disorders may lead to other disturbances in the normal functioning of the body, involving arms, legs, and even the nose.

Let us assume that you go to the grocery store. Arriving home, you unload the groceries on the doorstep, unlock the door, prop it open, and bend at the waist as you lift the heavy parcels again to bring them into the house. A few hours later you prepare dinner, spending a couple of hours on your feet. You notice that your back hurts and that there are small shooting pains running down your right leg. According to one chiropractor, this is the time to see a chiropractor. You may have the common "slipped disk."

Practitioners assert that through chiropractic "adjustment" this type of pain is easily relieved. Holistic practitioners require exercises after treatment to aid one in strengthening muscles so that they are able to remain in condition and withstand this type of strain. The chiropractor will also instruct the client to stoop when picking up heavy parcels. Most of the chiropractors with whom we talked believe that we all need to learn how to stand, sit, move objects, and maintain a healthy back.

Holistic chiropractors profess that this type of structural disorder can manifest itself functionally with defects either in body, mind, or spirit. A chiropractic healer is concerned with the effects and prevention of spinal disorders. For this reason, posture and physical fitness are the main emphasis of treatment. We have listed some ways one can check spine and posture alignment recommended by Dintenfass (1970):

Checklist for Spine and Posture Alignment

1. Does your head tilt to the right or left?
2. Does the middle of your neck curve?
3. Is one shoulder lower than the other?
4. Does one hip protrude farther forward than the other?
5. Is one hip higher than the other?
6. Can you move your head fully from left to right or forward and backward without difficulty?
7. Do you find it difficult to bend forward or backward from the waist?

If one can answer yes to any of these questions, chiropractors feel, a visit to a chiropractor for adjustment would be beneficial. The ACA will send interested consumers pamphlets, booklets, texts, and slide shows upon request.

There are essentially two types of chiropractors: the mixers and the straights. Mixers argue for the differential diagnosis and treatment of dis-ease. Straights locate, analyze, and correct subluxations, which in themselves are considered detrimental to health. The difference in the two is both one of goals or objectives and methods. Mixers are members of the American Chiropractic Association and by law are not allowed to advertise that they diagnose or treat dis-eases. The straights' professional organization is the International Chiropractor's Association. Straights only use manipulation or adjustment to clear the spine and nothing else. They restore the correct energy balance to the body, which they believe will then heal itself quite naturally. The mixers use many other techniques, such as nutrition, manipulation, psychotherapy, first aid, rehabilitation, water treatments, or any other "natural" method deemed necessary by the chiropractor. Neither the mixers nor straights prescribe drugs or surgery.

A holistic mixer recently told us that the conflict between the two schools of chiropractic is due to an overemphasis upon technique rather than a concern with a change in attitude by the healee. He feels that the healee's attitude is important because it is a motivating factor for igniting self-healing processes. In his words, "I have seen literally thousands of patients over the years, and I feel that most of them were relying solely upon me and my techniques to 'cure' them rather than a personal change to a holistic consciousness."

This statement implies that the two divisions of chiropractic are, from a holistic perspective, a false distinction based upon unwarranted assumptions. On the other hand, he maintains the viewpoint that spinal disorders do occur and should be prevented. The false distinction lies in the fact that both factions insist that:

1. Disease can show itself in any area of the body.
2. Natural measures should be taken to "treat" disease.
3. The individual is the key to the healing process.

From the turn of the century until the 1960s, chiropractors primarily served the elderly and needy in rural areas and those who could not afford osteopaths and physicians. However, during the 1960s the children of the more affluent upper middle class in cities began to visit chiropractors. Increased physical activity associated with the physical fitness movement and its related injuries also played a part in the growing role of chiropractors in modern life. We have interviewed many consumers with back problems, anxiety, and other disorders associated with stress as well as runners and other athletes who have made chiropractors an essential part of their lives.

We met a secretary who sits all day long unless her boss wants her to run errands. Even though she attempts to have proper posture, she "slumps" after a few hours in her chair. In order to circumvent this, she visits a chiropractor on a regular basis for spinal realignment. Her chiropractor functions to help her maintain a healthy back. She receives education from the practitioner concerned with improving posture and specific exercises for preventing the "slump." Without the reinforcement of the chiropractor, she believes that she would develop serious back problems. Be sure that you do not fall into the "trap" of excessive dependence upon a chiropractor. Return when you must. Otherwise listen to his or her advice and work to prevent back problems. Practitioners point out that this example is common to them. They recommend that consumers go when they have a problem and learn to prevent its recurrence.

It is estimated that on 5 to 10 percent of the chiropractic profession actually espouse the holistic philosophy in their daily practice. Though most of the literature we have received and the interviews we have conducted contradict this estimate (made by chiropractors), we think it is best for consumers to be made aware of it. Even if one has to visit several chiropractors before selecting a practitioner who implements the holistic philosophy into his or her practice, do it! Ask those you are considering if they include a holistic viewpoint and if they believe in the self-regulating aspects of the human body rather than an excessive reliance upon the techniques chiropractic utilizes to realign the spine. Also inquire as to the other aspects of the holistic philosophy outlined in the introduction to this book.Chiropractors are one of the most popular of the holistically oriented methods and as such deserve the attention of the consumer. However, there are many cases in which "rigorous scientific" training becomes a panacea for almost every ailment rather than a holistic method for health maintenance.

Type of Healing

Although chiropractors do not prescribe drugs, any number of diagnostic procedures may be employed to pinpoint the source of disorders. Some of these include orthopedic and neurologic examinations, X-ray examinations, observation, postural and spinal analysis, and in-depth interviews.

Chiropractors tell us that one of their basic beliefs is that "the greatest good for the patient" is the primary concern. The procedures and instruments used are standardized. The fact that chiropractors (mixers) make use of so many procedures, they maintain, is an advantage. An "extremely thorough" examination is supposed to allow the chiropractor to receive a total picture of the patient. The total picture is consistent with the goals of holistic methods and philosophy.

According to the ethics of chiropractors, you must either be treated or referred after an examination. As we have already mentioned, the profession today is attempting to establish itself by using the requirements of science. However, chiropractors say that they are willing to modify any of their procedures if it best serve the needs of the client. This includes working with physicians to design and implement a combined program of therapy.

Your posture has a bearing on work efficiency and comfort as well as resistance to some dis-eases and disabilities. Our bodies must be free from structural distortions in order to operate efficiently. The chiropractor maintains that he or she raises the efficiency level of the body to meet the day-to-day demands of life, thereby allowing the structural efficiency of the body's functions to take place naturally. During maximum efficiency, the bodily functions are in tune.

Many chiropractors declare that they can detect functional disturbances caused by irritated nerves long before symptoms appear. Thus, the preventive nature of chiropractic allows one to stabilize bodily operations and keep them in working order. Many mixers will attempt to be "scientific" in their approach, and most straights prefer to be known as scientists who only use the natural healing abilities of the body. Chiropractic, then, as a type of healing is considered to be natural with a recent emphasis upon the procedures of science.

Chiropractic is a natural type of healing due to the fact that these practitioners rely upon the self-regulating mechanisms of the body rather than drugs and surgery. So, though it is a standardized procedure, it avoids the use of external intervention in the body's natural processes. Of course, this field was founded before these techniques became as popular as they are today. Though many consumers will utilize chiropractic as an alternative to drugs and surgery, they may overlook the preventive aspects of the field at large.

Description of Healing Method

Holistic chiropractors usually begin their examinations with intensive interviews. The healer uses some of this interview to develop a comprehensive case record representative of the individual being examined. A physical examination, common to most health professions, is the next part of the procedure. After a physical, one is given a spinal and postural examination, which is a combination of X rays and/or "finger tip" examination.

Many clients have a simple problem that can be adjusted through manipulation. In other cases, such laboratory tests as blood tests or electrocardiograms may be needed. The use of many of these types of tests is dependent upon individual complaints or the health care plan the chiropractor feels fits your unique needs. Rarely are chemical tests required. Most testing cannot be furnished by the chiropractor. Consumers, then, must undergo testing elsewhere at an additional cost.

There are several major methods of treatment employed by chiropractors: chiropractic adjustment, nutritional advice or supplementation, physiotherapeutic methods to enhance the adjustments such as ultraviolet light, ultrasound, hydrotherapy, or foot stabilizers. In some cases, taping, strapping, or even braces may be used. Exercises are initiated in order to aid recovery and prevent future problems. In most chiropractic practices, exercise is an integral part of therapy. Holistic chiropractors assert that they are counselors as well as healers. He or she may counsel clients on diet, posture, life-style, mental and physical attitude, or occupational safety. Most counseling is focused on these areas rather than personal and spiritual concerns.

Another point to think about is that a conscientious chiropractor will tell his or her client exactly what is planned and how it will be accomplished. He or she will also describe the potential dangers involved. After explaining the procedures, the client is asked to sign a statement of informed consent, giving permission to proceed with the adjustments. Holistic practitioners report that the form is also employed as a contract between practitioner and patient to establish the responsibility of the parties to specific suggestions for health.

Upon arriving at the office of a holistic chiropractor, one often finds that the sign in front reads "Holistic Life Center" or "Chiropractic Health Center" rather than simply "Chiropractor." When you enter the office, you are told to fill out the customary forms that every physician has, with such information as your occupation, residence, spouse, emergency numbers, health insurance, and so on. You may be surprised to find that there is a statement at the bottom that says, "Each will pay according to their own abilities, unless insurance coverage is involved." Believe it or not, there are actually clinics that hold to this dictum and still remain solvent. One chiropractor told us that when one gives in this manner, one also receives. He and his partner had instituted this policy for little over a year and had found that it continued to pay off.

After filling out the form, you will be called to see the doctor and taken back to an examination room. If the chiropractor is a straight, your examination table will look much like a collection of boards joined together with some minor covering, as the table is usually divided into several sections that can be raised or lowered independently. If he or she is a mixer, the table may be a couch with cushions and may be curved in some manner. These couches also have sections that can be moved independently of each other for specific manipulations.

When a holistic chiropractor arrives, he or she will begin the examination with a personal interview, which we just mentioned, in order to develop a complete history of the problem. This includes any personal factors that may have contributed to it, such as inadequate posture, improper diet, or an attitude or consciousness focused upon dis-ease rather than health. This portion of the "treatment" is what many would call an initial counseling session. The chiropractor may prescribe increased vitamin intake or more rigorous daily exercise, or he or she may provide you with a course in correct posture.

After the preliminary counseling session, the holistic chiropractor will begin by realigning your back. If he or she is a mixer, other techniques, such as ultraviolet light or water therapy, may also be employed.

After treatment is completed, you may be asked to see other staff members for further suggestions or to experience other healing techniques. In some holistic clinics a masseuse and/or acupressure expert might provide additional therapy or make an appointment with you for further preventive treatments.

Diseases Treated

Recently, the Department of Health, Education and Welfare released the six leading causes of activity limitation in America (cited in *Consumer's Guide to Chiropractic Health Care*, 1977). They were as follows:

    13.2 percent heart conditions
    10.8 percent arthritis and rheumatism
     6.1 percent impairments of the back and spine
     5.6 percent impairments of lower extremities and hips
     3.7 percent asthma with or without hay fever
     3.6 percent mental and nervous conditions

The second, third, and fourth causes of limited activity are due to musculoskeletal disorders, which, practitioners feel, can be treated through chiropractic care. Other dis-eases associated with the musculoskeletal system are backaches, pain and spasms, headaches, arthritis, bursitis, disk syndrome, neutritis, low back pain, neuralgia, postural defects, sacroiliac pain, sciatica (affecting hip or hip nerves), spinal curvature, colds, fibrositis (excess fibrin in the blood), sports injuries, sprains and strains of joints and muscles, whiplash, noninfectious bronchitis, colitis, constipation, digestive disorders, hay fever, nervous disorders, dysmenorrhea (painful menstruation), and sinusitis. The average percentage of cases recovered or greatly improved from chiropractic care ranges from 73.3 to 93.3 percent (Dintenfass, 1970).

Duration of Treatment

The length of time one may have to remain under chiropractic care depends upon the nature and severity of the problem. Most therapy measures take at least six weeks to complete, but they may take as long as six months. There is a combination of treatments involved, which accounts for the lengthy period of time you have to spend under care. Additionally, holistic centers employ other therapy measures that require the expertise of other professionals. Chiropractors maintain that their success rate and client satisfaction, however, make this a minor point.

Adjustments make their relief known immediately, whereas other natural methods take longer to notice. The effects of exercises and nutritional restructuring, for example, may seem slow. Remember that exercises that are structured around the ailment are important in keeping the body toned and in proper (efficient) working order. Practitioners point out that nutritional recommendations also benefit the assimilation of energy, maintenance of health, and prevention of dis-ease. Nutrition is focused upon balanced meals, eating the correct mixtures of food, and eating while in the proper frame of mind. Furthermore, in many cases the chiropractor who is a mixer may suggest that you take vitamin or mineral supplements and/or herbs in addition to adequate nutritional intake. In most cases, these "natural" substances are contained in bottles on a separate shelf or in a separate room of the clinic or health center.

Cost Range

The cost of chiropractic care varies with the combination of treatments given, the individual's ability to pay, and the number of supporting staff members. Although it is advertised that chiropractors give workshops, we were unable to find any individual healers that do. Some clinics and colleges indicate they are willing to provide workshops if interest is expressed. The cost range for most chiropractic services follows:

Initial visit (without X rays)—$9 to $25

Examination (with X rays)—$35–$100 (complete X ray)
$25–$40 (sectional X ray)

Adjustments—$9–$25 (cheaper for senior citizens)

Laboratory testing—$25–$35 (single tests)
Laboratory testing is not provided by straights, and state licensing procedures may not allow other chiropractors to give these tests.

Follow-up visit—$9–$18 (cheaper for senior citizens)

Counseling—included in fees

Medicaments—included in fees
Some practitioners charge for supplementations.

Personal Responsibilities

Chiropractors maintain that there are three major reasons for vertebrae misalignment: lack of movement, sitting, and inadequate exercise. These can ruin health if they become unconscious life-style traits. Mental stressors that contribute to tension and nutritional deficits can also lead to subluxations. Your responsibility as a consumer is to make certain that these problems are overcome in your daily routine and/-or environment. This may only involve learning to sit correctly or walking a certain distance daily. However, if these are suggested by a chiropractor and are not implemented into daily activity, dis-ease can return.

A well-balanced diet is often recommended to consumers who visit a chiropractor. Whether this includes consumption of vitamins and/or minerals or simply adjusting vegetable intake, dietary suggestions play an important role in any holistic method. Professionals in this field report that most consumers neglect this aspect of total care, thereby neglecting the body as a whole. It is crucial that you assume the steps needed to incorporate correct nutritional habits if the body is to function to its optimum capacity.

Consumers will have to be aware of any symptoms that appear with structural and/or functional disorders even if they occur in parts of the body not necessarily associated with the spine. This is a precautionary measure to enable consumers to "spot" dis-ease before it occurs or to describe symptoms to the practitioner. If these are noticed, however, at the conclusion of chiropractic treatment, contact your practitioner.

Question all procedures. Not only will this keep you informed of what is being done to your body, it will also tell the inner portions of the body that you care about its functions. Although this may seem somewhat strange, practitioners point out that patients who show an interest in therapy actually facilitate the procedure. As consumers, the questioning of techniques can also provide you with a knowledge about possible solutions should a problem recur.

We must point out that consumers who wish to make use of holistic chiropractors investigate the practice of the chiropractor before agreeing to care.

As mentioned earlier, a chiropractor, straight or mixer, is not always holistic in practice. Be sure to get a description of the practitioner's general practice methods before making a trip to the office. Since chiropractors are licensed in all fifty states, contact the ICA or the ACA to find out if he or she is licensed in your particular state.

Informational Organizations

International Chiropractors Association
1901 L. Street, NW, Suite 800
Washington, D.C. 20036

American Chiropractic Association
1916 Wilson Boulevard
Arlington, VA 22201

Foundation for Chiropractic Education and Research
3209 Ingersoll Avenue, Suite 206
Des Moines, IA 50312

International Publishing Company
PO Box 2615
Littleton, CO 80122

Consistencies

1. Though chiropractors insist upon "rigorous scientific" procedures, they also believe that most of the body's healing power is self-regulating or natural. A combination of the scientific and natural is employed to provide the consumer with spinal adjustments and therapeutic adjuncts, life-style changes, attitudes, preventive nutrition, sanitation, and rehabilitation. Since both the physical and mental aspects of health are emphasized, this field claims to be consistent with the goals of the holistic model.

2. As with other holistic practitioners, chiropractors believe that individuals have the power to heal themselves and that the healer has the responsibility to motivate the patient. As mentioned earlier in the chapter, the most difficult client for a chiropractor is an apathetic one. Cooperation on the part of an active patient and faith in the healing process are crucial components of chiropractic care.

3. Chiropractors claim to have a valid alternative approach to healing. They have expanded their curriculum in recent years in order to include such subjects used in medical training as anatomy, biochemistry, and physiology. This has helped improve their status with the federal government. Their emphasis upon holism has also made their approach more popular among consumers.

4. Chiropractors believe that by unlocking human potential through the removal of spinal or nerve blockage, they open one of the major channels of human expression. Though this field does diagnose and treat dis-ease, it is consistent with the holistic principle that unlocking human potential provides consumers with a physical state consistent with health.

Inconsistencies

1. There are two acknowledged philosophies of chiropractic: the mixers and the straights. While this conflict is generally obscured from consumers, it involves basic contradictions in chiropractic principles. Straights feel that balance can only be attained through spinal adjustments and that "mixing" other procedures with spinal adjustment creates "unnatural" intervention. This is important because straights do not want the public to confuse them with chiropractors who are mixers. Second, mixers are defined as those who diagnose and treat dis-ease in a differential manner, whereas straights only analyze and correct subluxations. Legally, only physicians have the mandate to diagnose and treat dis-ease.

2. Though the medical profession (AMA) for years has claimed that chiropractors are "quacks," some doctors are now beginning to refer patients to them. Although we do not have any figures that tell us how many physicians feel that chiropractors are useful for certain problems, it is now a legitimate modality in the eyes of the Department of Health and Human Services. This fact alone does not make it inconsistent with the aims of holism, but there is a great deal of emphasis upon technique rather than upon innate healing potential. After all, spinal manipulation alone will not maintain well-being. Chiropractors insist that they have more to offer than holistic principles, since they claim to be a separate and distinct science. They are a specialty not duplicated by any of the other health professions. This type of professionalization, if not held in check, has the potential for leaving holism behind as an emphasis upon more specialization begins to fragment the view of the whole person.

3. There are at least seventeen colleges of chiropracty in the U.S., none of which are accredited by an independent association. Only eight are accredited by chiropractors themselves (Council on Chiropractic Education), while the rest are not (this includes one of the best known: Sherman in South Carolina). While chiropractic is becoming more legitimate, its "scientific" basis is not enough for full educational legitimacy. We wonder if part of the problem is that while it claims to be holistic, the overemphasis upon spinal manipulation is still seen by many as unscientific and opposed to a holistic philosophy of treatment. For example, many newspapers advertise free X rays, but holistically oriented practitioners maintain that indulgence by patients in X rays can be hazardous to health, since there is a link between radiation and cancer.

Sources To Read

American Chiropractic Association. "Consumer's Guide to Chiropractic Health Care" (pamphlet). Des Moines, IA: American Chiropractic Association, 1977.

Asher, Cecile. Postural Variations in Childhood. London: Butterworths, 1975.

Bach, Marcus. The Chiropractic Story. Los Angeles: DeVorss and Co., 1968.

Ballantine, Thomas H. "Will the Delivery of Health Care be Improved by the Use of Chiropractic Services?" New England Journal of Medicine. Vol. 286, 3, February, 1972, pp. 237 to 242.

Bolin, Darold E. The Philosophy of Chiropractic. Philadelphia: Dorrance and Co., 1974.

Consumer Reports. Chiropractors: Healers or Quacks? (Part I). Mt. Vernon, NY: Consumers Union of United States, 606–10, 1975.

Cowie, James, and **Roebuck, J.** An Ethnography of a Chiropractic Clinic. New York: Free Press, 1975.

Cyriax, James. Treatment by Manipulation, Massage and Injection. Baltimore: Williams and Wilkins, 1971.

Deimel, Diana. Vision Victory. Glendora, CA: Diana's Nutritional Center, 1972.

Dintenfass, Julius. Chiropractic: A Modern Way to Health. New York: Pyramid, 1970.

Feldenkrais, Moshe. Awareness through Movement: Health Exercises for Personal Growth. New York: Harper and Row, 1972.

Higley, Henry G. The Intervertebral Disk Syndrome. Des Moines, IA: American Chiropractic Association, 1965.

Jensen, Bernard. You Can Master Disease. Solana Beach, CA: Jensen's Nutrition and Health Products, 1974.

Kane, Robert L., et al. "Manipulating the Patient—A Comparison of the Effectiveness of Physicians and Chiropractic Care," The Lancet, June 29, 1974, pp. 1333–1336.

Larson, Leonard A., ed. Fitness, Health and Work Capacity. New York: Macmillan, 1974.

Levine, Mortimer. The Structural Approach to Chiropractic. New York: Comet Press, 1964.

Palmer, Bartlett Joseph. Shall Chiropractic Survive? Davenport, IA: Palmer School of Chiropractic, 1958.

Palmer, D. D. The Science, Art, and Philosophy of Chiropractic. Portland, OR: Portland Printing House, 1910.

Schafer, R. C. Chiropractic Health Care. Des Moines, IA: Foundation for Chiropractic Education and Research, 1977.

———. Chiropractic State of the Art. Des Moines, IA: American Chiropractic Association, 1976.

Schafer, R. C., ed. Basic Chiropractic Procedure Manual. Des Moines, IA: American Chiropractic Association, 1974.

Scofield, Arthur G. *Chiropractic: The Science of Specific Spinal Adjustment.* London: Thorsons, 1968.

Silverman, Milton, and **Lee, P. R.** *Pills, Profits and Politics.* Berkeley, CA: University of California Press, 1974.

Stoner, Fred. *The Eclectic Approach to Chiropractic.* Las Vegas, NV: F.L.S. Publishing Co., 1974.

Tansley, David, and **Baker, D., M.D.** *Radionics and the Subtle Anatomy of Man.* Rustington, Sussex, England: Health Science Press, 1972.

Thie, John, D. C. and **Marks, M.** *Touch for Health.* Los Angeles: DeVorss, 1973.

Wardwell, Walter I. "Chiropractic among the Healing Professions," *Journal of the American Chiropractic Association,* 1968, pp. 13–19.

White, Marjorie, and **Skipper, J. K.** "The Chiropractic Physician: A Study of Career Contingencies," *Journal of Health and Social Behavior,* 1971, pp. 300–312.

Wild, Patricia B. "Social Origins and Ideology of Chiropractors: An Empirical Study of the Socialization of the Chiropractic Student," *Sociological Symposium* 22 (1978): 33–54.

Wilk, Chester A. *Chiropractic Speaks Out.* Park Ridge, IL: Wilk Publishing, 1973.

7

MEDITATION

Definition

Meditative practices have been found in most ancient scriptures and among many so-called primitive sciences. The methods and techniques of meditation vary with each of those belief systems. Likewise, there are many definitions of meditation. Some of these definitions are as follows: to expand good feelings and experiences, to develop the heart, to meet God or ALL THAT IS, to look at the mind, to add meaning and value to life, to experience oneness, to heal and regulate the body, to attain nothingness, to increase self-confidence, and to focus attention. These are just a few of the definitions of meditation that we have collected in our research on the subject. When one looks at all of them, one major element emerges; they are holistic in that there is a definition for the spirit, the mind, the body, and the emotions.

We have been led to believe that only the most sacred of mystics can practice meditation. For example, shamans created a meditative atmosphere with ritualistic chants before administering a cure to their patients (Malinowski, 1925). Modern practitioners of this ancient art have begun to realize that the techniques used in meditation are actually very practical, thereby affording anyone a chance to attain these "sacred" attributes. However, only a chosen few were allowed to lead meditative ceremonies. So why all the secrecy? Experts tell us that if the masses had been aware of the method and techniques, those who "had the power" would not have been able to maintain control of the situation (Kluckholm, 1944; Weber, 1963; Yinger, 1969).

The contribution of meditation to holism is twofold. First, meditative techniques allow you to relax, the obvious benefit being that you are able to release stress and face other challenges with a clear mind. Second, meditation asks that you question your actions, feelings, and self in order to come up with the underlying reasons for these actions and feelings. In other words, the self-examination process seems to release (give you) more control over your life. You learn that society does not "run your life" but that you do and that you can actually be in control of what happens to you.

Meditation, like acupuncture, is concerned with what meditators believe to be the inner energy of which everything is composed. Within most of the theories of meditation, energy has three elements that fluctuate and need to be balanced. These energy elements are the physical structure through which energy flows; the breath that energy moves through, and the subtle energy (usually associated with mental energy), which is elusive.

These energies are connected to the four centers of the body: (1) The body itself—its physical structure—is related to the navel center; (2) the breath is related to the throat; (3) the mind, or subtle energy, is related to the head; and (4) all are contained within the heart.

> When the three elements or energies move through the centers, certain conditions or attitudes are produced—physical sickness, mental blockages, emotional troubles . . . or feelings of lightness, radiance, and total openness. The basic patterns of our physical functioning both determine and are determined by how the energy flows through these very subtle centers. Whenever we are sick, unbalanced, or have negative feelings, these are always indicated by the patterns, the movement, and the essence of energy within the body. Therefore, in order to be healthy we should learn how to balance our body, breath, and mind [Tulku, 1976].

All meditation is healing in that it vasodilates, decreases pulse, respiration, and blood pressure. There is no difference between meditation and healing meditation. The purpose of this chapter, then, is to describe its function within holistic health, not write a treatise on its spiritual nature.

It should be obvious from what we have already presented that there are several methods of meditation. We cannot advocate any one approach as being more valid than another. However, there has been some evidence on TM and yoga that demonstrates that the individual can learn to control blood pressure, heartbeat, and other bodily functions. An individual practitioner may be more inclined toward one.

Objectively speaking, each of the methods has a particular goal. One may be better suited to your personal needs than another. Holistic practitioners of this art believe that any of the methods can be used to create a healthier state of mind. They also maintain that the benefits of meditation include both the ability to deal with yourself in private and the ability to deal with others. An added advantage of meditation is that it does not require a teacher or practitioner in order to be healing. In other words, consumers can make use of meditation on their own for self-healing.

After interviewing several holistic meditators, we compiled the following illustration of practical application. Imagine that you are a schoolteacher with your life centered around an academic routine. Each morning you wake up, get dressed, eat breakfast, go to school, and teach six classes with thirty or more students a day. After school there are many other activities in which you must engage, such as planning and organizing lessons for the next day, attending faculty meetings and parent conferences, and going home where another part of your life awaits you with an entirely different set of responsibilities. Upon arriving home, you probably feel exhausted and personally disorganized. You have spent your entire day living for others rather than for yourself. This pattern leads to a situation where you may begin to feel a lack of personal accomplishment. Most teachers will continue their day in the same routinized fashion: eating dinner, having drinks, doing a little work for school, watching TV, taking a shower, and returning to bed for "rest" before another day.

Here we notice several characteristics of what holistic practitioners have termed ill health: routine rarely changed because of a feeling of necessity, emotional strain resulting from social intercourse with both students and colleagues, feelings of disorganization because one has done "too much," and a period of inactivity after returning home that is defined as "relaxation" before the drudgery of the next day. Peace of mind is missing from this routine. Meditators insist that regular practice of meditation can change this feeling. Though you may feel that alloting the time for meditation will only add more "fuel to the fire" by giving you another activity to fit into an already busy schedule, it may actually change the conception of your routine, making it appear more spontaneous than before. This internal change in your perception allows your emotions to rest so that your day becomes less demanding emotionally.

Meditation provides the private time that meditators believe is required for one to feel more organized. If you take fifteen or twenty minutes for afternoon meditation, they believe that you will feel more relaxed in the evening. You will not feel so rushed before beginning your day. If something exciting comes up or friends "pop in" for a visit, you will be able to enjoy them with genuine feelings of joy rather than "senseless" interruption. About now you might be asking yourself, "All of this with a little meditation?" Meditators reply affirmatively and feel that you can have more if you wish.

Research indicates that two fifteen-minute periods of meditation a day are equivalent to a two-hour nap. The brain produces *alpha waves* during meditation, signifying a deep state of relaxation but not loss of consciousness (Brown, 1977). This "nap" lowers blood pressure and helps prevent asthma, sinusitis, migraines, ulcers, insomnia, and alcoholism and allows one to avoid cigarettes and have an improved outlook on life. One problem with this research is that the body centers of subtle energy we just mentioned have yet to be discovered. However, the effects themselves are valid, reliable, and real.

Sincere holists emphasize that meditation is not exclusive or magical—it is a practical means for enhancing personal well-being. Many meditators maintain that consumers have the wrong idea about meditation—that is, that meditation is mysterious and difficult. In reality, meditation is easy. This image, meditators feel, has been fostered by popular conceptions of meditation drawn from the mass media and experience with pseudoreligious organizations. A legitimate method of meditation is free, is possible without a religious organization, and only takes courage and self-discipline. They ask that one set stereotypes aside and view it as a preventive tool for improving state of mind and preventing dis-ease.

Type of Healing

Meditation is a natural healing method. No drugs are given to help you; no herbs are given to initiate a meditative state of mind. You are on your own. One has to be self-motivated by a desire to balance inner energies. Of course, holistic meditators believe that it is a major step for taking responsibility for your health. One is taught to "hold on to your mind" so that you can look into it and discover what is there and why.

As just stated, "balance" is the key to meditation. This ability to balance bodily energies begins by observing your own thoughts and feelings while learning to examine the interrelationship between your mind and body. Your thoughts and feelings may be stronger in some areas than in others, so you are taught to examine the area and *intensity* of the feeling.

Since there are so many methods used to accomplish balance, perhaps the most meaningful methods are the simplest. For example, relaxation and visualization are extremely useful for the "average" consumer wishing to experiment with meditation. One often wonders just how this procedure can produce such a healthful feeling. It is best described as a process. Most teachers of meditation maintain that to experience feelings of relaxation and focused attention is revitalizing. Why not try this simple relaxation visualization exercise for yourself? We have compiled several procedures into the following technique: Take your phone off the hook, stop your chores, and sit or lie in a comfortable position. Tighten all the muscles in your body and inhale deeply. Exhale slowly and completely relax constricted muscles. Check to make sure that your eyebrows, mouth, and shoulders are relaxed. Inhale and exhale deeply while counting to twenty-five.

In your mind picture a country road in October. You are walking down the road slowly. The birds are singing. They fly overhead and you look up to catch the sight of two crows chasing each other across the treetops. The wild flowers are blowing in the cool autumn wind. A butterfly moves to another flower because a black and yellow bee has moved into his territory. Grasshoppers jump in the bush as you walk along the road.

The sun feels warm in the October breeze. You see the sun's reflection on the ground as it creates a path of diamonds. Trees rustle and leaves fall in front of you. The sweet gum trees are red and the sassafras trees are yellow. An oak tree has still some green leaves, and the pines are all green. The leaves seem translucent in the sunlight. It's so colorful and bright that you feel overwhelmed.

You come to a small stream with a sturdy old wooden bridge. The rocks are polished by swirling water as tiny fish are dashing from rock to rock. The shadows of trees dance across the water. The water reflects rainbows on the backs of the leaves overhanging the stream. As you walk across the bridge, you watch the shadows move across the water. The green moss on the rocks makes a small waterfall and the water sounds soothing as it rushes under the bridge. Lush growth next to the stream sways with the wind. The smell of damp earth and crisp air engulfs you as you stare at the clear blue sky. Crickets, frogs, and birds sing to you as you stand in the autumn hues of gold and rust. You are happy and relaxed.

Slowly open your eyes. Notice how relaxed and refreshed you feel. Your body feels warm; you are rested. Emctionally, you are calm.

You may envision any scene for relaxation, any situation you wish to change, any idea you want to expand, or any dis-ease you need to correct. Including all the details, and using your imagination, you simply construct the scene the way you wish it to be. An illness may then be transformed into health, a problem may be viewed as a solution, an idea may be an invention, dreaded activities may become challenges.

Of course, this is the simplest form of meditation and is similar to self-hypnosis. It is called relaxation and/or visualization, but it clearly represents the ease and balance that can be creatively used to heal the spirit, mind, and body. Advocates of this process believe that by learning to focus attention, you can become aware of internal and external characteristics affecting your balance—that is, your state of ease.

Since practitioners and physicians who use meditation have no "formal organization" through which one can make contact, many healers practicing meditative techniques will be found in institutions directed toward psychology, group therapy, transpersonal psychology schools, and awareness centers. In this context we can also mention autogenic therapy. Autogenic therapy is a combination of hypnosis, meditation, and deep relaxation techniques.

Meditation, therefore, is a primary factor in *autogenic therapy*. One is taught exercises, visualizations, sensuality, imagery, and other techniques that are said to enhance the meditative state. Autogenic therapy can be specifically oriented toward illnesses because a professional therapist (usually a psychologist) is constantly working with you. In this way, guidance is always provided and changes can be constantly monitored.

Though there is someone to help you in autogenic therapy, you are usually your own healer in meditation. Autogenic therapy is psychological, whereas meditation presents the challenge of gaining strength through will power. Autogenic therapy may be better suited to your needs if you require external discipline in order to accomplish goals.

Description of Healing Methods

One may have to search for a practitioner who uses meditation. The chances that your healer will be a physician will be slight. In fact, meditation does not require the skill or intervention of a physician. Most of the meditative techniques can be self- or group-taught. And, even if you are fortunate enough to find a physician who does teach meditation, the healer still relies upon you to help yourself, thereby providing the best of both worlds.

Physicians who recommend meditation often use biofeedback, a popular tool used to aid clients in learning and achieving a state of relaxation for the specific treatment of ailments. The term *biofeedback* was developed because biological information generated by clients was "fed" back to them (Brown, 1977). Dr. and Mrs. Simonton and James Creighton (1978) have used another offshoot of meditation—guided imagery (see Chapter 14)—along with changed beliefs about cancer to improve malignancies.

Relaxation is not as easy as it sounds. You need to become aware of the relationship between mind and body. For example, upon noticing a flow of images, concepts, or thoughts, you may feel that you are in an unbalanced state. The mind is always active and if one cuts off experience, a chain reaction is started in the body. So, one is taught to begin by observing your own thoughts and feelings.

Physical and mental exercises are often used to prepare you for meditation as a meditative method. Physical exercises tone your body. Yoga is an example of this process. Most meditators believe that exercises create vital energy for use and distribution within the body. Just as in yoga, it is believed that exercises align and balance the body. Mental exercises may be employed to describe relationships between yourself and your society, your mind and a diseased organ, what you are doing and what you *want* to be doing, or ease and dis-ease within your body at different times and in different situations.

Since you and your practitioner will have to decide which methods best suit your personal needs, we will briefly describe some of the different approaches in the following paragraphs. Most of these categories have been combined from Ayra (1974), Blofeld (1977), Stevens (1974), Tulku (1977), and others.

Concentration meditation is somewhat different from visualization in that you concentrate upon your dis-ease, your thoughts, or your feelings. Concentration will allow your conceptions to expand and dissolve. This method is especially good for those who feel that others control their lives, and it can help one rid oneself of negative thoughts and feelings. The problem is supposed to disappear because you have faced it, expanded upon it, explored it, and no longer find any use for it.

Mantra meditation is also used quite frequently. Mantras have to do with sounds. The mystery associated with mantras is only symbolic. Mantras can be the soothing sound of rushing water, a musical tone, or a nonsensical word. The sound itself must be soothing and healing to you. Some believe that you can actually make up your own sound. It is constantly repeated in your mind in conjunction with rhythmic breathing while you are in a relaxed state. Constant repetition is supposed to break up normal thought patterns and allow new or different patterns to enter your mind. The exact manner in which the use of a mantra quiets the mind has yet to be explained. Users of this method feel that once one has allowed new thoughts to enter, old thoughts no longer seem important. However, as far as we know, experimental evidence of this belief has not been presented.

Analytical meditation is a much longer process and is usually explored by an interested individual or a group with this specific goal in mind. Here people are asked to do such things as count the number of thoughts that go through their mind in one hour. After you have done this for several days, you try to find the relationships between your inner and outer selves. You are supposed to learn to observe how these two facets of the whole personality work together to create your world by noting conflicting thoughts. The goal of this type of meditation is to "know thyself." The meditators teach that thoughts should be your own and not imposed upon you by parents or others' perceptions of you; you should see yourself as you are, not as others say you are. You learn to say no to the things you have always wanted to say no to and yes to those things that are really important to you.

Another method used in meditation therapy is *experimental meditation*. Here one learns to observe experiences and to study them. None of the experiences are labeled or judged. Once again, you study the conflicting experiences, discovering how they are either similar or different, and eventually find out how your experiences promote or inhibit health.

You can tell from the brief descriptions of these types of meditation that, as meditators tell us, there is nothing so mysterious about it when you understand what to expect. They believe that it has very practical, everyday applications to stress and stress-related situations. Therapists teach short relaxation techniques to ease stress before stress dis-eases you. For example, when you are emotionally taxed, many suggest that you sit quietly and breathe softly and gently. Do not pay attention to your emotions; just follow your breath and its rhythm. This short exercise can be both calming and healing.

These types represent some of the most popular methods used in meditation. There are many other methods that are also self-actualizing. Generally, breathing and relaxation are taught first. When totally relaxed, the body should experience a warm feeling. Relaxation can be increased with physical massage, and many may have to use massage to ensure relaxation. These exercises are supposed to revitalize and balance the body, so that one is not growing in just one area and neglecting another.

If dietary counseling is available, it is used to increase consumption of fruits, vegetables, fish, grains, and nuts. Most healers also recommend decreased intake of fats, meats, white flour products, and sugar. If your healer uses nutrition along with meditation to enhance relaxation and prevent stress, diet will be monitored with each consecutive visit. Monitoring nutritional balance allows you to become aware of mental and physical changes experienced when eating certain foods. Tightening of the muscles following a cup of coffee or sugar snacks is supposed to indicate that caffeine and sugar create an imbalance in your vital energies.

This self-examination system, according to meditators, has the ability to bring about changes in those who use it. Beliefs that are constructed around dis-ease, negative thoughts, and unconditioned bodies may be restructured to include a healthy attitude and responsibility for your thoughts and actions. These changes, we are told, often act as a catalyst promoting health before it is actualized and giving one goals to attain during treatment.

We met with a great deal of enthusiasm when researching meditation. Many claimed that it changed their entire lives. Others felt that they were transformed into being more loving, patient, and considerate of others. But, the comment we received most often was, "I learned about myself, what my self is." And their health? Well, they just "weren't that sick anymore." These seemingly "indirect" effects of meditation upon health are astonishing to most and surprising to many we have interviewed. Perhaps when they "let go" of dis-ease, they actually forget what it is like and do not wish to experience illness as they used to do. Though there have not been any long-range studies of the effects of meditation upon physical health, the correlation between meditation and well-being is, for now, simply a question of personal experience with it and faith that it will occur. Thus, though it may be a self-fulfilling prophecy, many satisfied meditators feel healthier because of its application. We do know, as we have mentioned, that there is a relationship between meditation and blood pressure, increased alpha waves and skin resistance. A lower metabolism, an increase in energy and ability to deal with daily routine, a decrease in psychosomatic reactions to stress, a lower systolic blood pressure, and less drug abuse are some other beneficial traits reported by researchers of meditation (Hoffman, et. al., 1982; Benson, 1976; Wallace, 1970).

How to Know You're Meditating

You need to recognize when you are meditating so that you won't be expecting something else. As you start meditating, thoughts may be buzzing through your head. Let these thoughts go. Outside noises will seem louder but not necessarily disturbing. You can hear the rhythms of your body: your breath, your heartbeat. You become detached from your surroundings in that you have warm feelings in your arms and legs and may not feel the surface upon which you are resting. When everything "becomes blank," that is, your sense of time is lost or the thoughts going through your mind have stopped, you have transcended. Upon waking, you have the feeling of heightened sensibility. You are as relaxed as if you had slept for six hours. There also seems to be an increased amount of energy.

The combined link to spirit, mind, and body, according to most meditators, makes meditation a valuable therapeutic healing method. There is not supposed to be a separation between you and your world, as many of us have been taught to think of meditators' life-style. Diet, exercise, and meditation are the basis of therapy. This is accessible to consumers because there are many "how to meditate" books available. It does not require a great deal of time to master the procedure, just the capacity to experience it on a daily basis.

Disease Treated

Meditation will not cure any dis-eases. It has been successfully used to treat high blood pressure, cancer, migraines, sinus problems, asthma, stress, diabetes, stomach ulcers, sexual problems, sleep problems, constipation, arthritis, such addictions as smoking habit, alcohol, and obesity as well as cramps and such emotional states as insecurity, fear, or anxiety.

Duration of Treatment

The length of treatment varies with the type of meditation you are using. It will also depend upon whether or not you are using techniques that are self-actualizing. Self-actualizing methods take longer because treatment will not only center on illness but will include therapy on your world, your beliefs about your world, how you relate to that world, and what you want to do with your life. Your actions must concur with the beliefs you hold; consequently, this process takes time. Some of the self-actualizing methods of meditation are contemplation, passive attention, absorption, discipline, the way of self-surrender or expression, and the negative way. These treatments will often take three to six months to heal a dis-ease, but many profess that self-actualization is a lifetime process.

Other meditative techniques such as relaxation, visualization, biofeedback, autogenic therapy, immobility, concentration, spontaneous movement, and not doing take somewhat less time to treat dis-ease. By using one of these methods the duration of your treatment is usually one to five months. Most meditative healers recommend that you continue meditation as a preventive measure, even without your healer. This allows the body to maintain balance, thereby preventing future dis-ease.

Physicians who use meditation will also vary. But be wary of those who only treat your symptoms. Meditation is a more comprehensive program, asking that one use meditation to treat the underlying causes of dis-ease. Here, the duration of treatment varies more with the specific ailment than any other factor. In many cases, once your symptoms disappear, you will not be asked to take preventive measures through meditation, nutrition, and exercise. In other words, there is no real way to tell exactly how long it will take to feel the effects of meditation on a specific ailment. Instead of expecting to be cured of a specific dis-ease in a short period of time, consumers must learn to be patient with their health. Once meditation is mastered and practiced daily, meditators point out, you will begin to believe that it is miraculous because one no longer falls prey to the chronic ailments, such as colds and high blood pressure, that once plagued your very existence. Rather, you will not seem to become ill as often as before you started meditating.

Cost Range

The cost of meditative healing therapy is as illusive as contacting a healer in the field. If you use a physician, the cost of meditation is combined with his or her fee. But, if you go to a group for training in meditation (which most probably does not specifically include healing per se), your fee is considerably higher. Hopefully, the following will give you some idea of the variations of cost for meditation. Holistic healers recommend that you purchase a book to learn how to meditate rather than taking a course, although that may require more self-discipline.

Initial visit (with a physician)—$25–$50
Initial visit (with a meditative healer)—$40–$75
Follow-up visit (with a physician)—$20–$30
Follow-up visit (with a meditative healer)—$25–$30
Counseling (diet and exercise)—included with both
Meditation courses (one week to six to eight weeks)—$50–$200
Healing institutions (residency)—$250–$500 (per week, including room and board)

Personal Responsibility

Professionals using meditation request that you discipline yourself daily. This discipline is self-imposed in diet, exercise, and meditation. Each of these are to be incorporated into daily or weekly routine. Dietary requirements vary from healer to healer. Some prefer fresh fruits and vegetables, little meat, whole grains, and dairy products. Others are not oriented toward "freshness" so much as the quantity of foods you ingest. You are expected to eat on a regular basis (three to six meals a day), not gorge yourself for two days and eat skimpy the other five. Your diet shows your body that homeostasis is possible, enabling it to function with some regularity. The same is true of exercise, since the body becomes positively "addicted" to a daily pattern of physical activity.

One also has to decide which meditative position is most comfortable. Most professionals prefer you use a sitting position because you may fall asleep while lying down. One position does not necessarily work better than another. Your choice should be based upon your own standards of comfort.

Meditative healers will express that you must have faith in meditation and your own ability to meditate and help yourself. According to these experts, disbelief in the process and its potentials will block your healing energies. Meditation strengthens the will. Disbelief is action against the will. The fact that you are willing to try to heal yourself acts as a catalyst for your body's potentials.

In meditative healing you are accountable to yourself. Your physician or healer may get you started, but you must continue to meditate in order to keep your body healthy and your energies balanced. Needless to say, this time will also give your emotions a well-deserved rest from the constant stimulation they received each day. Body toning exercises will also be your responsibility. Remember, if you only follow through with part of the therapy, you will not grow equally in spirit, mind, and body. You will only receive part of the cure. Overemphasis on one part is as bad as not following through with any of them.

From our viewpoint meditation is work. It is not easy to construct a detailed scene, focus on a thought until it expands, or relax totally for twenty minutes. You must be patient and remember that you are learning to release yourself. It has been hidden for a long time. You have been caught up in specific habitual ways of thinking, acting, and feeling for years. Now, you must learn to undo all these mental habits.

Meditation, taken by itself, may not cure. You, as healee, must comply with all the changes you will have to make. This entails following a good diet, taking time for yourself, exercising out of doors, and changing harmful habits and life-styles. You may find that it is easier to go to a "conventional" healer if you do not have your mind made up to be responsible for your own well-being before trying this modality.

Informational Organizations

Himalayan Institute
Route 1 Box 88
Honesdale, PA 18431

Foundation for Inner Peace
PO Box 635E
Tiburon, CA 94920

We found it very difficult to contact professionals that use meditative healing. There is no professional organization that can help you besides groups of meditators such as TM. But these groups do not focus on healing. The Himalayan Institute is very reliable and will help one find a professional in your area. Many physicians will be glad to look around for you and try to obtain the name of a reliable professional. Don't be afraid to ask your doctor. He or she would rather you go to someone that you feel will do the job than not seek treatment at all.

Consistencies

1. The definitions of meditative healing outlined in this chapter emphasize the role of spirit and mind in healing. Whereas some approaches to meditation (such as yoga) also emphasize the body, this is not always the case. In any event, meditators teach that a balance between body and mind is essential for healing to occur.

2. Meditators maintain that the process has taught them about their feelings and changed their lives. It appears to be one of the safest techniques for self-realization available to the public and can be used for both discovering the self and establishing mental health.

3. The "natural high" fostered by meditation and the prohibition of narcotic highs by meditators implies that it is one possible solution to the drug problem in modern society. Andrew Weil (1972), a physician, suggests that meditation can eventually replace the need for drug use (also see Forrester, 1971).

4. Since establishing balance is a fundamental assumption of meditative therapy, it offers a spiritual avenue that has the potential of promoting tolerance of diversity in society because of a mutual interdependence or balance. Persons with "balanced" minds and bodies may wish to expand these beliefs to include their enemies as well as their friends. Meditators teach that inner peace can lead to global peace, since the external world is only a reflection of the internal one.

5. Meditation offers many methods to the consumer. Each of these have different aims. Anyone, then, should be able to find one to suit his or her own needs. If the choices are too difficult, then consumers might try to develop their own methods for achieving the meditative state on a daily basis.

Inconsistencies

1. Meditation has been associated with mysticism throughout history. This "shroud of secrecy" has kept many away from it, since they have perceived it as sacred and unattainable for the average person. Meditation must be demystified before its more practical use in healing can be accomplished successfully. Some meditative organizations have ignored the body in favor of spiritual "cults." The reputable meditative healer must allow for free will from the consumer and attempt to construct an individualized program. If your healer includes these elements, you will in good hands. If not, do not be afraid to go elsewhere.

2. Meditative therapy has more of a mind-spirit orientation than some methods and more of a body-mind orientation than others. Consumers may find it necessary to use the techniques that feel comfortable and also stress the balance between mind, spirit, emotions, and body.

3. Meditative healers may not be aware of the role of proper nutrition and exercise in their treatments. Taken alone, meditation is not a cure-all for any ailment. Be sure and use a meditative technique that includes all three: nutrition, exercise, and meditative awareness.

4. There is no general listing of meditative healers available from professional organizations. This means that there is no way to verify questions about the distribution and use of meditation within medicine at this time. The emergent nature of this technique is a major reason for its inaccessibility.

5. Excessive amounts of meditation can lead to "burnout." The technique requires a great deal of discipline on a daily basis. If you go to sleep or neglect other duties and just meditate, you are not using it properly for health maintenance.

Sources to Read

Akhilananda, Swami. *Mental Health and Hindu Psychology.* New York: Harper and Row, 1951.

Arya, Usharbudh. *Superconscious Meditation.* Prospect Heights, IL: Himalayan International Institute of Yoga, 1974.

Assagioli, Roberto, M.D. *Psychosynthesis.* New York: Viking, 1971.

Bailey, Alice. *From Intellect to Intuition.* New York: Lucis, 1972.

Baker, Douglas, M.D. *Meditation: Theory and Practice.* Little Elephant, Kentish Land, Essendon, Herts, England: By the Author, 1975.

Bauman, E., et al. *The Holistic Health Handbook.* Berkeley, CA: And/Or Press, 1978.

Benson, Herbert, M.D. *The Relaxation Response.* New York: William Morrow, 1976.

Blofeld, John. *Mantras: Sacred Words of Power.* Boulder, CO: Shambhala; 1977; New York: Dutton, 1977.

Brown, Barbara. *Stress and the Art of Biofeedback.* New York: Harper and Row, 1977.

Budhananda, Swami. *Mind and Its Control.* Hollywood, CA: Vedanta, 1972.

Chang, Chung-Yuan. *Creativity and Taoism.* New York: Harper and Row, 1975.

Conze, Edward. *Buddhist Meditation.* London: Allen and Unwin, 1968.

Curtis, Adela M. *Of Meditation and Health.* London: School of Silence, 1910.

Downing, George. *Massage and Meditation.* New York: Random House, 1974.

Forrester, Jay W. "Counterintuitive Behavior of Social Systems," in *Technology Review* 73, no. 2 (1971), p. 3.

French, A. P.; Smith, A. C.; and **Ingalls, P. O.** "Transcendental Meditation, Altered Reality Testing, and Behavioral Change: A Case Report," *Journal of Nervous and Mental Disease* 1 (1975): 55–58.

Gersten, D. J. "Meditation As an Adjunct to Medical Psychiatric Treatment," *American Journal of Psychiatry*, 135, no. 5 (May 1978), pp. 598–599.

Goldsmith, Joel S. *The Art of Meditation.* New York: Harper and Row, 1957.

Govinda, Lama A. *Creative Meditation and Multidimensional Consciousness.* Wheaton, IL: Theosophical Publishing House, 1976.

Green, E. E.; Green, A. M.; and **Walters, E. D.** "Voluntary Control of Inner States: Psychological and Physiological," *Journal of Transpersonal Psychology* 2, no. 1 (1970), pp. 1–26.

Gutwrith, Samuel W. *How to Free Yourself from Nervous Tension: An Exact Scientific Method for Relaxing Body and Mind.* Chicago: Regnery, 1955.

Hanson, Virginia, ed. *Approaches to Meditation.* Wheaton, IL: Theosophical Publishing House, 1973.

Harvey, Bill. *Mind Magic*, 3d ed. New York: Irvington Press, 1980.

Hills, Christopher. *Nuclear Evolution: Discovery of the Rainbow Body.* Boulder Creek, CA: University of Trees, 1977.

Hoffman, John W., et. al., "Reduced Sympathetic Nervous System Responsivity Associated with the Relaxation Response," *Science 215* (January 8, 1982): 190–92.

Humphreys, Christmas. *Concentration and Meditation: A Manual of Mind Development.* Baltimore: Penguin, 1973.

Jacobson, E. *Anxiety and Tension Control.* Philadelphia: Lippincott, 1964.

Kluckholm, Clyde. *Navaho Witchcraft.* Cambridge: Harvard University Press, 1944.

Kroll, Una. *The Healing Potential of Transcendental Meditation.* Atlanta: John Knox, 1974.

LeShan, Lawrence. *How to Meditate: A Guide to Self-Discovery.* Boston: Little Brown, 1974.

Malinowski, Bronislaw. "Magic, Science and Religion," in *Science, Religion and Reality.* ed. J. Needham. New York: Macmillan, 1925.

Masters, Roy. *How Your Mind Can Keep You Well: A Book about the Ancient Science of Meditation.* Los Angeles: Foundation Books, 1971.

Meares, A. "Regression of Cancer after Intensive Meditation," *Australian Medical Journal* 2 (July 31, 1976): 194.

Null, Gary. *Biofeedback, Fasting, and Meditation.* New York: Pyramid, 1974.

Oates, R. M., Jr., ed. *Celebrating the Dawn.* New York: Putnam's, 1976.

Paramananda, Swami. *Concentration and Meditation.* Boston: Vedanta, 1974.

Pelletier, Kenneth. *Mind as Healer, Mind as Slayer: A Holistic Approach to Preventing Stress Disorders.* New York: Delacorte, 1977.

Progoff, Ira. *The Practice of Process Meditation: The Intensive Journal Way to Spiritual Experience.* New York: Dialogue House, 1980.

Puryear, H. B., Ph.D., and **Thurston, M., Ph.D.** *Meditation and the Mind of Man,* rev. ed. Virginia Beach, VA: ARE Press, 1975.

Rama, Swami, and **Ajaya, Swami.** *Emotion to Englightenment.* Glenview, IL: Himalayan International Institute of Yoga, 1976.

Ramakrishna Vedanta Center. *Meditation.* London: R.V.C., 1972.

Samuels, Mike, M.D., and **Samuels, N.** *Seeing with the Mind's Eye: The History, Techniques and Uses of Visualization.* New York: Random House, 1975.

Sanford, J.A. *Healing and Wholeness.* New York: Paulist Press, 1977.

Saraydarian, Haroutiun. *Science of Meditation.* Agoura, CA: Unity Press, 1972.

Schultz, J. H., and **Luthe, W.** *Autogenic Training.* New York: Greene and Stratton, 1959.

Shames, Richard, M.D., and **Stern, C.** *Healing with Mind Power.* Emmaus, PA: Rodale Press, 1980.

Simonton, O. Carl, M.D.; Matthews-Simonton, Stephanie; and **Creighton, James.**
Getting Well Again. Los Angeles: J. P. Tarcher, 1978.

Speeth, Kathleen Riordan, Ph.D. *The Gurdjieff Work.* Berkeley, CA: And/Or Press, 1976.

Stevens, Edward. *An Introduction to Oriental Mysticism.* New York: Paulist Press, 1974.

Suzuki, Shunryu. *Zen Mind, Beginner's Mind: Informal Talks on Meditation and Practice.* New York: Weatherhill, 1972.

Truch, S. *The TM Technique and the Art of Learning.* Toronto: Lester and Orpen, 1977.

Trungpa, Chogyam. *Meditation in Action.* Berkeley, CA: Shambhala, 1970.

Tulku, Tarthang. *Gesture of Balance: A Guide to Awareness, Self-Healing, and Meditation.* Emeryville, CA: Dharma Press, 1976.

——. *Kum Nye Relaxation.* Emeryville, CA: Dharma Press, 1977.

Wallace, Robert K. *Physiological Effects of Transcendental Meditation.* Los Angeles: Students International Meditation Society, 1970.

Weber, Max. *The Sociology of Religion.* Boston: Beacon Press, 1963.

Weil, Andrew. *The Natural Mind.* Boston: Houghton Mifflin, 1973.

White, John, ed. *What is Meditation?* Garden City, NY: Doubleday, 1974.

Yinger, J. Milton. *Religion, Society and the Individual.* Toronto, Canada: Macmillan, 1969.

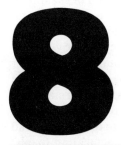

SPIRITUAL HEALING

Definition

Throughout history most classical civilizations have placed a great emphasis upon what we now call *spiritual*, or *faith*, *healing*. The power of kings and queens was based, in part, upon their spiritual beliefs. According to sociologists and historians, people presumed that royal monarchs possessed two bodies: one mortal or private and one immortal or public. The latter was translucent or ephemeral and was considered to be divine. It could not be seen or communicated with by ordinary means. Instead, the divine royalty was perceived to be skilled in advising, guiding, and planning for the welfare of their subjects. Furthermore, though the mortal personalities of these monarchs died, their public bodies lived on in the memories and experiences of the kingdom and led to certain ostentatious burial practices as well as the custom of power being passed down through the royal family.

These conceptions were as important to political power as democracy and legislatures are today. One may question how a king, owner of all land (or kingdom), ruler of the people, as well as judge, jury, and prosecutor, could be respected in this manner. One answer is that the monarch's public body contained the "healing touch." Those who were afflicted, ill, or poverty stricken would line up on special occasions to receive the divine touch of the king or queen. Though we really have no idea how many of these subjects were cured, histories of Western civilization contain documented cases of miraculous cures very similar to the miracles performed by Christ in the New Testament and by other historical religious personages. Thus, though there were most certainly many unsuccessful cures, the tradition of the "king's touch" remained. As democracy emerged, the practice gradually died out. Leaders were elected and then defeated in political contests that were totally removed from any sort of divine inspiration. Consequently, the "healing touch" gradually filtered into society and the church.

When the scientific method began to dominate cultural thought, faith healers became associated with the church, where natural, unobservable laws permitted the "miracle" of healing when scientific medicine failed. Christ had become the model of a person, divinely inspired, who had healed through the power of God, and that energy thus became known as "God power." It flowed through the hands of special people who were believed to have a special "connection" with it. These practices revived the classical affirmations of two bodies simultaneously working together for a worldly purpose and the healing of those who were hopelessly ill.

It is important, at the outset, to realize that spiritual healers claim that they do not feel they are the gatekeepers of God power. They acknowledge that everyone has spiritual gifts and that these may be developed in many ways, one of which is to heal. Anyone who seeks healing is asked to make their mind and heart receptive through meditation and/or prayer. Healers in the spiritual field feel that they are merely instruments through which the power of God flows. Healing is accomplished through touch or laying on of hands, faith in God, God power, prayer, songs, or meditation and visualization. Spiritual healers contend that God supplies an unlimited supply of life force or universal energies. Each individual, according to this logic, contains life energies that may at some point be obstructed, thereby causing dis-ease. The healer "tunes in" to the universal supply of energy and, like a conductor, channels this energy into the body from which energy has been depleted.

There are several kinds of spiritual healers, and some of them overlap with those in the psychic field. Many of their abilities, beliefs, and characteristics of their healing overlap. For instance, spiritualists most often have *psi abilities* (extrasensory perception, telekinesis, and mediumship) in addition to healing competencies. The spiritual healer, however, attributes his or her abilities to God, Christ, the Holy Spirit, or all three, whereas the psychic healer does not necessarily assert a religious doctrine, although as far as we have been able to determine, both claim to make use of identical energies. The Reverend Canon William V. Rauscher is one of the leading researchers in the spiritual field and has devoted many years to both the church and the paranormal. His work on both psychic and spiritual healers has led him most accurately to state, "If a saint hears angelic voices, it is a spiritual experience" (1975).

Spiritualists believe that miracles demonstrate natural laws. These laws are universal "givens," the major tenet being that of cause and effect of a "balanced" life. However, this simple cause-and-effect relationship places great emphasis upon belief and faith in the healing power of God as well as adherence to religious doctrine. Through faith and ethical behavior, it is believed, prayer supplies the healer with God power. This process builds a trancelike state in which God's energy is activated before healing can take place. It is this "miracle" of healing that has inspired many people with religious ideals for most of recorded history.

We found that spiritual healers have termed their treatments as supplementary to orthodox medical practices. A legitimate healer will not ask that one abandon medicine, drug therapy, or a physician's care. With the exception of absent healings, where there is no face-to-face contact with the healee, most spiritual healers will not make appointments with anyone who has not previously seen a doctor unless all of the doctor's treatments have failed. Although there have been cases of healing "miracles" in degenerative or the final stages of dis-ease, healers prefer to see a person before these last stages because of a higher rate of cure.

Spiritualist practitioners point out that dis-ease occurs in response to thoughts and actions. That is, thoughts and actions are not consistent (in harmony) with the natural flux of all that surrounds us. Legitimate spiritual healers *do not* believe that dis-ease is caused because of sin, that you cannot be healed if you do not have faith in God, or that you should give up all medical treatments and substitute faith for physicians. Should a healer place these conditions upon healing, our recommendation is to find another one or be prepared to join a religious cult.

We found this the hardest area in which to judge fraudulent aspects of healing occupations. Clearly, there are many frauds associated with faith healing. But, even those who are found to be charlatans have clients who claim to have been healed. Most practitioners point out that the belief in the practice and power of God by the healee, accompanied by the belief that healer can heal, is the reason behind these cures. Fraudulent healings often take place in overt settings. For example, there are many so-called healings taking place on television screens and in tents across rural America. The audience may be "primed" by a couple of "staged" healings before it actually participates in the healing process.

Thus there are a few precautions that can be taken by any consumer interested in spiritual healing.

1. Research the practitioner as well as those that work for him or her.
2. Obtain the names and contact others who have made use of this healer. Question the effectiveness of the treatment, the cost, and the length of time the cure lasts. Legitimate spiritual healers are more than happy to share the names of previous clients.
3. Settle for a healer who takes time to document his or her work. These are often personal case histories requested by the healer that describe a "before" and "after" picture of the healee.
4. For effective cures the faith of the healee should be equal to that of the healer. Faith in a practitioner's ability also facilitates healing.
5. Ask a family member or friend for support. Cures often leave one whose beliefs are not reinforced outside of the healing setting.
6. Do not touch a healer during laying on of hands. In such cases it is possible to cause a reversal of the healing process.

We can only tell you to use careful consideration when choosing a healer. Use your head and don't rely on a "good line." Spiritual healers, for the most part, live according to religious beliefs and should therefore seek to exemplify their tenets. If a healer talks religion and acts like a sailor, you certainly want to find someone who is more consistent.

Some of the famous spiritual healers of our times include such names as Edgar Cayce and Ambrose and Olga Worrall. These healers have countless claims and documents from those who have benefited from their help. Each of these healers attributed his or her abilities to God. They promote the idea that, through His grace the ability to heal is channeled through them so that they may help others. Science has been unable to interpret these types of healers or explain the abilities shown by them. It is the intangibility of the spiritual plane, its ethereal forms and mystique that have made many scientists utter, "When in doubt, leave it out." However, even though spiritual healing may seem ambiguous and fraudulent, genuine cures are a legitimate part of the record.

Type of Healing

Spiritual healing is a natural method of healing based upon religion. Spiritual practitioners hold to the belief that dis-ease displays itself in the body, but it originates in the spiritual realm. Healing, thereby, must take place in the spiritual stratum in order to heal a body's physical or emotional manifestations (symbols) of disease. With the use of visualization, meditation, and, most important, prayer, spiritual "medicine" is delivered to the system. Visualization includes seeing the part as whole, watching a smoothly functioning system, creating a new picture of health. Meditation soothes a system, points out emotional and spiritual problems, offers renewed vitality through relaxation, and is recommended as reinforcement for the "healing touch" by nurse Delores Krieger (1979).

Prayer promotes faith and individual strength. It is with prayer that a healee asks for help from all of God's energies. Building faith in self aids healings as well as establishes faith in the strength and "knowing" within that an answer will come or a way will be shown.

Some spiritual healers will rely upon religious beliefs and incantations to initiate the healing process. These may be Bible meditations, songs, or prayers. When you meet a healer on a one-to-one basis, prayer and Bible meditation establishes the healing mood. Prayer and/or meditation lasts from ten to fifteen minutes before a combined, concentrated visualization or the laying on of hands occurs. In both cases, healees report feeling energy enter from the direction of the practitioner. Prayer groups create a religious service and include the singing of hymns along with prayer and meditation lasting about thirty minutes. The group then visualizes healing energy entering the body to fill it with self-healing strength. Prayer group services continue until all who have asked for help have been included in prayers.

Many practitioners in this area say that the two worlds of allopathic medicine and spiritualism interact and are complementary. They claim that both fields concentrate upon healing, both provide care for specific areas, both acknowledge the other, both make use of prayer, both recognize that physical systems are interconnected with spiritual ones and therefore must interact, and both allow for miracles. If the two worlds are indeed complementary, why, then, do we not see practicing spiritualists in hospitals and clinics?

We have learned of some scientific evidence that supports spiritualists' claims of laying on of hands and concentrating energy, most of which is reported in the next chapter, on psychic healing. Science, as yet, has been unable to prove or disprove the validity of the entire field of spiritual healing. Nor can scientists explain the abilities shown by some spiritual healers. A number of researchers have attributed some of the successes of these healers to their manner of producing a trancelike state in the healee or to the relationship developed with the healee during the healing. For instance, empathy, bodily contact, and a warmth expressed by the healers in this field might help produce a healing environment that facilitates faith in God and individual healing traits, which in turn inspire expectations that one will be healed.

Some practitioners of faith healing are eager to point out that faith often activates an individual's self-healing God power. One's faith may be strengthened in the knowledge that twice the help is available to heal, that of God and that of the practitioner. But, there are preventive measures one may take to increase individual faith and to maintain well-being through God. More than likely, some of these might benefit each of us as general guides for living.

Guidelines for Spiritual Well-Being

1. Respect your body and treat it as a holy place.
2. Believe that you are related to everything in the universe.
3. Pray or meditate for yourself and others at least five minutes a day.
4. Love all others.
5. "Do unto others as you would have them do unto you."
6. Help one another along the path of life.

Another spiritual method that may be of use to consumers involves a form of visualization. This consists of visualizing a body as it was before the dis-ease. Harold Sherman, the famous psychic and spiritual researcher, who recommends this method, says, "Things first have to occur in mind before they can happen in body. Thus, when the perfect pattern of the body has been replaced in mind, activated by sufficient faith, this pattern has to be reflected and reproduced, in whole or in part, in the physical side of life" (Sherman, 1972).

The majority of persons termed spiritual healers are associated with some form of organized religion. They usually adhere to seven major tenets that support faith in God, man, and soul. Power to heal is accepted as a gift from God to be used to help others. Fred Archer (1966), editor of *Psychic News* and researcher of spiritual phenomena, tells us that spiritualists have not yet gathered around any specific creed. He found that spiritualists may hold the following tenets, but these will be interpreted individually according to doctrine.

1. The Fatherhood of God.
2. The Brotherhood of man.
3. The Communion of Spirits, and the Ministry of Angels.
4. The continuous existence of the human soul.

5. Personal responsibility.
6. Compensation and retribution hereafter for all the good and evil deeds on earth.
7. Eternal progress open to every human soul.

Interestingly enough, in spite of solid reliance upon God and other external forces, personal responsibility is of great importance to spiritual healers. Perhaps this is because of the importance of faith. It goes without saying that all spiritual healers are grounded in faith. How the faith is used, to exploit or help, is another matter, not covered in this book. We must, however, caution consumers about "blind faith." "Blind faith" is accepting every suggestion, comment, and experience without thinking about or examining them or the consequences they may bring. Consumers should be objectively critical enough to know when a healer is "handing you a line." For example, spiritual healers should not *insist* on using mediumship or seances to heal. Although the two may not be contradictory, many people have been fooled by magic.

Description of Healing Method

Spiritual healers attuned to the power of God make use of laying on of hands, group prayer, prayer, and visualization and/or meditation as well as absent healings. One or more of these are employed in conjunction with the Scriptures, sacraments of the church, and faith. With the exception of absent healing most of these techniques are part of a "rituallike" ceremony that prepares the healer and the healee for energy from God. This formality can be compared with an abbreviated church service that establishes a healing environment.

As we examine each of the methods employed here, notice that there are only minute differences between them. That is, most ceremonial observances are identical except that they are group ventures rather than one-on-one encounters. It is likely that gatherings for spiritual healings will take place in a private home rather than a church or meeting hall. Thus, prayer groups often rotate meeting sites among participating members, whereas individual practitioners are usually found at one specific location, although it may be secret so as to avoid trouble with the law.

The healing atmosphere, as established earlier, is fostered by praying, meditating, and/or Scripture readings. An individual or a group will be led in these activities by the healer and his or her assistants. Before prayers it is suggested that a donation be made, but it is stressed that money is not necessary in order for healing to take place. After the collection everyone is asked to pray for divine healing aid. Each is asked to step into a separate room to be treated by the practitioner while the others wait their turn. After each person has been treated, the group of healees is blessed.

Laying on of hands, sometimes known as therapeutic touch, is the most publicized method of healing used by spiritual healers. Researchers of laying-on-of-hands techniques (most notably Dr. Thelma Moss at UCLA) note that Kirlian photography reveals the hands of healers emanating a large amount of energy, or aura, when compared with the average hand. In this method the healer can either touch a body on the forehead and shoulder or hold his or her hands two to four inches from the body. One is as effective as the other and depends upon the practitioner's personal style. A heatlike energy is released by the healer and is often felt by the healee as a mild electrical discharge or warmth. The entire healing process of laying on of hands usually takes from seven to ten minutes. Sometimes there is a need for several touching treatments, but, in most cases, relief is felt instantaneously. We would like to remind all potential clients that a healer who uses laying on of hands cannot be touched while he or she is transferring energy because a reversal of that energy can cause a "backfire," leaving a "short-circuited" healer.

Prayer groups operate throughout most states and are contacted through and affiliated with many different religious denominations. They are composed of any number of interested people and use the methods of prayer, visualization, song, and meditation. Individuals pray for those who have requested healing aid, made a donation, or require spiritual help. These groups are not limited to healing in that they replenish energy to those with any type of need and, for this reason, should not be confused with absent healing groups. Although most groups accept outside participation, one does not have to attend in order to receive help.

Absent healing is performed by spiritualist associations and groups and can be differentiated from prayer groups by the use of the word *spiritual* or *spiritualist* in its name. Their gatherings may congregate around one spiritual healer who is the "leader" of the group, or all members may be considered healers, group members combining energies to heal others.

Consumers mail healing requests to the group. Although not necessary, absent healers prefer to work with a photo so that "images and energies" of the healee can be more easily attained in the mind's eye. Absent healing groups schedule their meetings at a particular time on a specific day each week. Those who are thinking about absent healing groups must understand that consumer participation is not encouraged. On the other hand, consumers wary of spiritual healing may find absent healing an ideal path for their needs because of the lack of their actual presence.

Consumers who make use of absent healing participate by scheduling quiet time to meditate, pray, and relax during the group's scheduled healing time. Healees are asked to meditate upon God's energy filling the body, to pray for strength, and to relax so that the healing energy can enter their bodies. Absent healing groups point out that this procedure greatly facilitates healing action. A few clients have felt a warmth enter their body during participation with the group, but this cannot necessarily be attributed to the group. Again, donations for services are not required but are appreciated.

If one prefers an individual practitioner and cannot find one, most spiritual groups will offer referral services. It is possible to purchase a list of names and addresses from the American Spiritual Healing Association or the National Spiritualist Association of Churches, whose addresses are enclosed under "Informational Organizations." A letter or phone call will ensure that the practitioner is available. Consumers are asked to make a "prayer" or "love" donation before services of groups or practitioners. There are a few individuals, however, who do not accept donations.

Diseases Treated

According to spiritual healers, God can cure any dis-ease. With this in mind, we have listed below the diseases treated by spiritual healers. Our list is not comprehensive but it will list the most common ailments reported by representatives of this group: headaches, blindness, deafness, palsy, epilepsy, back problems, cancer, kidney ailment and stones, ulcers, nervousness, neuritis, crippling arthritis, emphysema, bronchitis, skin dis-eases, gallstones, angina, cataracts, tumors.

Duration of Treatment

Most spiritual healers will tell you that the degree of success of healing is dependent upon the nature of the dis-ease. We realize that this is very open ended, broad, and vague as well as being true of any method of healing. Ridding a body of symptoms is one thing, whereas healing the spiritual aspects, or roots of the dis-ease, is quite another. Prayer, songs, meditation, and/or visualization are employed to focus the consciousness of the healer and healee. It is said that if your faith in God, faith in the healer, and faith in your own ability to heal is strong enough, a cure will be immediate. Spiritual healers sometimes attribute healing of nonbelievers to the fact that God power and God's love is available to all.

The number of treatments thought to be necessary is dependent upon several factors: severity, length of the dis-ease, family support, and beliefs in and relationship with healers. Spiritualists report that most clients receive two to twelve treatments of laying on of hands, taking several months in the case of serious disease.

There are also questions as to the endurance of spiritual cures. Many clients report that after leaving the healer for a period of time, the cure wears off. This occurs over a short period of time (five to twenty-one days). In some cases, cures reverse themselves almost immediately. Our research can only speculate as to the reasons for these occurrences. Stanley Krippner and Alberto Villoldo (1976) present the idea that the world view and belief systems of the healer are left behind by the healee once healing is completed. When the client returns home, he or she may not have the beliefs—that is, the cure—reinforced by family and/or friends. Spiritualists intimate that the healee's own body can take over or that another visit with the healer may be required in order for the cure to be effective. It is our speculation that there may also be a problem of relatives and friends in accepting the fact that an "unconventional" healer may have succeeded where a conventional healer failed.

We suggest that anyone who plans to see a spiritual healer ask for support from the whole family, a family member, or a friend before, during, and after the visit. This allows one to feel more at ease about the experience as well as reinforcing the cure's effects. Of course, it makes sense to choose a supporter who has similar beliefs and one who is comfortable with religious beliefs and this type of healing potential so that the process will feel more natural.

Cost Range

Free to $25

Personal Responsibilities

There are several responsibilities placed upon a consumer who decides to try spiritual healing. You must first have employed treatments provided by medical physicians before visiting a healer in this field. Spiritual practitioners do not wish to have any conflicts with organized medicine which might possibly befall them if you do not see a physician first. They feel that medicine and spiritual healing can work hand in hand to cure dis-ease. It is important to mention the fact that many conventional orthodox physicians are religious whether by definition, oath, occupation, or experience. It is possible that your physician may know a spiritual healer or someone to contact. If not he or she may at least be willing to try to visualize a cure with you, as mentioned earlier. If you do not feel close enough to a physician to ask his or her help, be honest and mention that you plan to see a spiritual healer. Your plans to make use of another type of healer may well open the door to aforementioned knowledge and more interest in your case.

Absent healing and prayer groups schedule healing sessions at particular times during one or two days a week. Remember that a snapshot increases the groups' ability to reach you, so don't forget to include one with the request. Make sure you are aware of the times for prayer so that you can relax and focus your attention on the healing process.

Individual healers, on the other hand, request that you phone or write for an appointment because their services are scheduled in advance. Many healers are members of absent healing groups or volunteer their services in other areas. If you just dropped in, flew in, or drove over, your healer might be busy with other healings or activities, and money would have been wasted (when the whole situation could have been avoided).

As we have previously mentioned, the experience will be more satisfying if a healer is chosen according to religious faith, similar beliefs, or past healings and reputation. A person of the Baptist faith may be offended by the wording in a prayer performed by a rabbi. A companion can facilitate the process after visiting a healer by adding support about the healing experience, helping others understand, and reinforcing the beliefs shared by those involved.

After you have visited with a healer you may want to have "backup" support from your family and or friend(s) at home. One obvious benefit of this is that all these people will be focused on your getting well. This works on the same principle as the Native American celebration of wellness described in Chapter 10. Social networks can provide assistance in numerous ways besides just talking with you about your experience or your dis-ease.

Some of you may seek to practice self-healing either in conjunction with a spiritual healer or alone. For those interested in such a procedure, we included the following exercise, paraphrased from Harold Sherman (1972)—a five-minute self-regulating plan for spiritual healing:

> Relax your body totally and place your attention on All That Is or the God Power. Ask yourself to balance your spirit, mind and body. Concentrate on these and let other thoughts go by. Pray for those in need. Ask the God Power to aid you in selecting and acting on those activities which will produce the greatest good for you and those in your world.

It should be evident by now that your most important responsibility in this method of healing is to examine in detail the techniques employed by spiritual healers. Begin your investigation by interviewing those who have already received services in order to determine if there is any sleight of hand or other fraudulent practices. Question assistants about the procedure used during the healing ceremony. Read over the measures taken by mediums to defraud others in the next chapter on psychic healing. Safeguard personal information when talking with a specific healer or his or her associates. Do not carry personal items into the healing setting. Recognize the fact that this method has been one of the primary areas of deception in holistic healing. We will summarize our conclusions regarding spiritual healers when we describe the consistencies and inconsistencies of this modality with the philosophy of holism.

Finally, remember that in spite of your skepticism and critical examination, the development of faith is the most crucial factor. Obviously, if you lack religious feelings and beliefs, another healing method would be more helpful. On the other hand, if you are "not a particularly religious person," we feel that the personal responsibilities just presented can aid in "building the faith." The investigative procedure outlined, designed to make you take on the role of detective or sleuth, will bring you into contact with the subject and the people or groups who should reassure you if you have personal misgivings. Remember this warning: Do not expect to be healed until you have completed your investigation.

Informational Organizations

We have to admit that spiritual healers are the most helpful and generous with information in understanding the principles of their practice. Enclose a self-addressed stamped envelope for easy return mail, and any of the organizations below will help you select a spiritual healer or absentee healing group that will suit your individual needs.

Stow Memorial Foundation
Mrs. Evelyn Muse
1104 Susan Drive
Edinburg, TX 78539

American Spiritual Healing Association
PO Box 1189
6 Bridle Path Circle
Framingham, MA 01701

National Spiritualist Association of Churches
PO Box 128
Cassadaga, FL 32706

Unity School of Christianity
Unity Village, MO 64065

Prayer groups are available through most religious denominations. Ministers of the selected religion will be able to give you information regarding these.

Consistencies

1. Spiritual healing coincides with the holistic philosophy in "the spiritual realm" as holism seeks to heal mind, body, emotions, and spirit. In other words, by considering the spirit as essential for well-being, spiritual healing seeks to broaden modern medicine, just as the holistic philosophy proposes to do.

2. Faith in God is the major personal responsibility required by spiritual healers. Therefore, a basic concept of holism, faith in well-being, is included even if in a somewhat convoluted form. The belief in clearing channels for the God power to work through you is a part of this consistency and is very similar to the idea of a vital force contained in most of the holistic modalities described in this book.

3. Spiritual healers base their curative process upon the natural laws of cause and effect as well as harmony with others and with nature. This is also consistent with the classical philosophies of holism. However, as described in an inconsistency, the notion appears to be antiquated when compared with modern syntheses of science and religion, which expound on these ideas to their fullest extent through the use of the term *multidimensionality*.

4. Spiritual healers work in cooperation with modern medicine and seek to incorporate those called to this occupation into the modern hospital system in order to aid physicians. This trend is consistent with the philosophy of holism in that modern practitioners of holistic modalities do not deny the importance of conventional medicine. Instead, they maintain that is it not enough, as faith and human understanding of spiritual factors and their relationship to dis-ease are both necessary and constructive.

5. Though spiritualists contain many contradictions, we are of the opinion that they are consistent with the holistic ideal of opening new vistas or frontiers of knowledge for modern science. Scientific experiments, then, are necessary to prevent fraud and aid consumers in their use of the valuable element of the spirit in the healing process.

Inconsistencies

1. Spiritual healing is only partially consistent with the philosophy of holistic healing, since nutritional practices, life-style counseling, and plans for personal action designed by the healer (in consultation with the healee) in order to facilitate total well-being are neglected. This lack of multidimensionality, therefore, is a major inconsistency of spiritualists.

2. As we researched these healers, we realized that there are many important contradictions contained in their methods. One of the most common is the use of "ringers" who "fake" the healing process in the emotional atmosphere of their ceremonies. We have interviewed some who were obvious frauds and used their personal charisma to become quite wealthy because they formed nonprofit organizations and skimmed money from the thousands of dollars collected at healing revivals.

3. Many practitioners require copies of previous tests before consumers can be accepted as clients, yet knowledge of the client's previous diagnosis is strictly forbidden by most healers as interfering with the healer's view of the body and is generally believed to be unnecessary. This is not consistent with holism, since most holists believe in maintenance of low-cost treatment. The money required for copies of diagnostic tests might be prohibitive for many consumers.

4. Spiritual healing is a natural method of healing based upon religion, yet most claim that God can heal regardless of previous beliefs and religious experiences. Reliance upon external forces rather than the self is inconsistent with holism and yet is quite consistent with allopathic medicine, where individuals are oftentimes perceived as the victims rather than the creators of symptoms. While we realize that these issues are complex and we can offer no ultimate answer here, we can say that both internal and external forces are dynamically interrelated. Healing should not be based upon superstition or the belief in an external force but upon faith in one's self to maintain well-being.

5. While spiritual healers are most often, though not always, associated with some type of organized religion, it should be emphasized that few of these religions support spiritual healing except under unique circumstances. For instance, some Old Testament prophets, Christ, and certain saints are still believed to have performed miracle cures. Yet some religionists emphasize that those cases are 1 in 10,000. Thus, most religions side with science and oppose spiritual healing, which means that within the religious camp there are as many contradictions and anomalies as in any other field of endeavor. The spiritual elements of holism, however, do not necessarily proceed from religious organizations or spiritual healing, rather from personal investigation and fulfillment of one's spiritual side in an individualized, nondogmatic manner.

Sources to Read

Archer, Fred. *Exploring the Psychic World.* New York: William Morrow, 1966.

Bach, Marcus. *The Power of Total Living.* New York: Dodd, Mead, 1977.

Barbanell, Maurice. *This Is Spiritualism.* London: Herbert Jenkens, 1959.

Cerutti, E. *Olga Worrall: Mystic with the Healing Hands.* New York: Harper and Row, 1975.

Cooke, Ivan. *Healing: By the Spirit.* Hampshire, England: White Eagle Publishing Trust, 1955.

Daily Word. Unity Village, MO: Unity School of Christianity.

De Ropp, Robert S. *The Master Game.* New York: Dell, 1974.

Dicks, R. *Toward Health and Wholeness.* New York: Macmillan, 1960.

Edmunds, Simion. *Spiritualism: A Critical Survey.* London: The Aquarian Press, 1966.

Edmunds, Tudor H., and associates, ed. *Some Unrecognized Factors in Medicine.* Wheaton, IL: Theosophical Publishing House, 1976.

Edwards, Harry. *Guide to the Understanding and Practice of Spiritual Healing.* Surrey, England: Spiritual Healing Sanctuary, 1974.

Frank, J. *Persuasion and Healing.* New York: Schocken, 1974.

Frankl, V. *The Doctor and the Soul.* New York: Knopf, 1957.

Fremenatle, Anne. *The Protestant Mystics.* Boston: Little, Brown, 1964.

Garrett, Eileen J. *Awareness.* New York: Helix Press, 1943.

――――. *Beyond the Five Senses.* Philadelphia: Lippincott, 1957.

Gaskin, Ina May. *Spiritual Midwifery.* Summertown, TN: Book Publishing Co., 1977.

Geismar, Maxwell. *Mark Twain: An American Prophet.* Boston, Mass.: Houghton Mifflin, 1970.

Guardini, Ramano. *Prayer in Practice.* New York: Pantheon, 1957.

Hall, Manly P. *Healing: The Divine Art.* Los Angeles: Philosophical Research Society, 1944.

Hammond, Sally. *We Are All Healers.* New York: Harper and Row, 1973.

Haynes, Reneè. "Miraculous and Paranormal Healing," *Parapsychology Review.* Vol. 8, 5, September–October: pp. 25–28.

Hollander, Annete, M.D. *How to Help Your Child Have a Spiritual Life: Inner Development with or without Organized Religion.* New York: A & W Publishing, 1980.

Hutschmecker, A. *The Will to Live.* New York: Crowell, 1953.

Ikin, A. Graham. *Studies in Spiritual Healing.* London: The World Fellowship Press for the Churches Fellowship, 1968.

Isreal, Martin. *Healing and the Spirit.* London: Churches Fellowship for Psychical and Spiritual Students, 1972.

――――. *Summons to Life: The Search for Identity through the Spiritual.* London: Hodder and Stoughton, 1974.

Jackson, Herbert T. *The Spirit Rappers.* Garden City, NY: Doubleday, 1972.

Jayne, W. A. *The Healing Gods of Ancient Civilizations.* New York: University Books, 1962.

Kiev, A., ed. *Magic, Faith, and Healing.* New York: Macmillan, 1964.

Kimmell, Jo. *Steps to Prayer Power.* Nashville, TN: Abingdon Press, 1972.

Krieger, Delores, Ph.D., R.N. *The Therapeutic Touch: How to Use Your Hands to Help or to Heal.* Englewood Cliffs, NJ: Prentice-Hall, 1979.

Krippner, Stanley, and **Villoldo, Alberto.** *The Realms of Healing.* Millbrae, CA: Celestial Arts, 1976.

Kruger, Helen. *Other Healers Other Cures.* New York: Bobbs Merrill, 1974.

Kuhlman, Kathryn. *God Can Do It Again.* New York: Pyramid Family Library, 1969.

Long, Max Freedom. *The Secret Science behind Miracles.* Santa Monica, CA: De Vorss, 1948.

———. *The Secret Science at Work.* Santa Monica, CA: De Vorss, 1953.

McHargue, Georgess. *Fact, Frauds, and Phantasms: A Survey of the Spiritualist Movement.* Garden City, NY: Doubleday, 1972.

Melton, J. Gordon. *A Reader's Guide to the Church's Ministry of Healing.* Evanston, IL: The Academy of Religion and Psychical Research, 1973.

Montgomery, Ruth. *A Gift of Prophecy.* New York: William Morrow, 1965.

———. *Here and Hereafter.* New York: Fawcett, 1977.

Moss, Thelma. "Radiation Field Photography," *Psychic Magazine,* July 1972, p. 50.

Nolen, William A. *A Doctor in Search of a Miracle.* New York: Random House, 1974.

Oursler, W. *The Healing Power of Faith.* New York: Hawthorn Books, 1957.

Paramananda, Swami. *Spiritual Healing.* Boston: Vedanta, 1975.

Parente, Pascal P. *Beyond Space, A Book about the Angels.* Rockford, IL: Tan Books and Publishers, Inc., 1973.

Parker, William R., and **St. Johns, Elaine.** *Prayer Can Change Your Life.* Englewood Cliffs, NJ: Prentice-Hall, 1957.

Ponder, Catherine. *The Dynamic Laws of Healing.* Marina Del Rey, CA: De Vorss, 1972.

———. *Dynamic Laws of Prosperity.* West Nyack, NY: Parker, 1962.

Powell, A. *The Etheric Double.* Wheaton, IL: Theosophical Publishing House, 1969.

Powers, Thomas E. *First Questions on the Life of the Spirit.* New York: Harper and Brothers, 1959.

Rauscher, Canon William V., and **Spraggett, Allen.** *The Spiritual Frontier.* Garden City, NY: Doubleday, 1975.

Rose, L. *Faith Healing.* Baltimore: Penguin, 1971.

Sanford, John A. *Healing and Wholeness.* New York: Paulist Press, 1977.

Sechrist, Elsie. *Meditation—Gateway to Light.* Virginia Beach, VA: ARE Press, 1972.

Sherman, Harold. *Your Power to Heal.* New York: Harper and Row, 1972.

Shoemaker, Samuel M. *With the Holy Spirit and With Fire.* New York: Harper and Brothers, 1960.

Spraggett, Allen, and **Rauscher, William V.** *The Psychic Mafia.* New York: Harper and Row, 1975.

Spiritual Community Guide. San Rafael, CA: Science Publishers, 1976.

Steiner, Rudolf. *Spiritual Science and Medicine.* London: Rudolf Steiner Press, 1948.

————. *The Philosophy of Spiritual Activity: Fundamentals of a Modern View of the World.* London: Steiner Books, 1980.

The Theosophical Research Centre. *The Mystery of Healing.* Wheaton: Theosophical Publishing House, 1968.

Thie, John, D.C., and **Marks, M.** *Touch for Health.* Los Angeles: De Vorss, 1973.

Van Vliet, Cornelius J. *The Coiled Serpent: Conservation and Transmutation of Reproductive Energy.* Los Angeles: De Vorss, 1959.

Von Reichenback, Karl. *Researches on Magnetism . . . in Relation to the Vital Force.* Secaucus, NJ: University Books, 1974.

Westlake, Aubrey T., M.D. *The Pattern of Health: A Search for a Greater Understanding of the Life Force in Health and Disease.* Boulder, CO: Shambhala, 1973.

Worrall, Ambrose, and **Worrall, Olga**. *Gift of Healing.* New York: Harper and Row, 1975.

Young, R. K., and **Meiburg, A. L.** *Spiritual Therapy.* New York: Harper and Brothers, 1960.

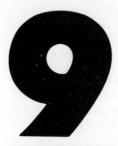

PSYCHIC HEALING

Definition

The history of psychic healing has been cloaked in controversy. *Psi phenomena* are, indeed, strangely exciting and offer almost unimaginable possibilities for the future of healing. Throughout history only dowsing can be labeled as the type of psi activity that was legitimated by society. Christopher Bird, in a recent book, has shown some very practical uses of dowsing by the Standard Oil Company. Even though homing pigeons have "sensed" their way back home and dogs have found their owners after they have moved hundreds of miles away, scientists, as a general rule, believe that human beings do not have this same type of "ability." Consequently, psychic healing has been thought of as only an "occult" silence.

When it comes to the subject of psi activity or psychic healers, there is often so much left unexplained that there is nothing left to explain! As we shall see, science proves it and rejects it. One might say, then, that psi power has healing tendencies, yet it does not heal every dis-ease or every person. For we have been told that logical processes can interfere with receiving psychic information, and so can concentration. Because psi happens when one is relaxed and it happens casually, it cannot be touched or seen.

There are basically four major kinds of psychic phenomena, excluding, of course, spiritual healing, which can also be considered a form of psi activity (see Chapter 8). *Precognition* is the receiving of information about the past, present, or future that could not have been obtained in such ways as reading or watching a TV show. *Clairvoyance* is acquiring information about objects or events without help from the known senses. *Telepathy* is communication between minds as information is passed from one person to another. The ability to move objects at a distance is known as *psychokinesis*. The *healing process* as accomplished by psychics rids the body of dis-ease when there is no medical, psychological, or physical way to explain its disappearance.

Within psychic healing, practitioners tell us that the body consists of different energies, energy patterns, or energy centers. One psychic describes this energy as existing in subtle bodies that interact with one another. The bodies are the *astral body*, the *etheric body*, and the *mental body*. The astral body is seen as emotional colors, and it is said that healers can read the colors projected by the physical body as well as emotional states related to the intensity (or lack of it) in these colors. For example, an emotional problem that relates to a dis-ease may be seen by a psychic healer as a dark area in the colors of the astral body.

The etheric body is responsible for the flow of "life energy" into the physical body. Some describe it as a force field that protects the body from dis-ease when one is healthy. Etheric bodies respond to the astral and mental bodies and reflect problems in the physical body. There can be deficits or excesses of this type of energy. An example of this might be one who feels like physical energy is drained after returning from a depressing visit or one who possesses an extra vitality that can be "given" to others when in a good mood.

From the psychic point of view, individuals are seen as part of the universe. The universe is seen as containing all living entities. Life is viewed as an opportunity to build and strengthen character and spirit. Dis-ease slows and, in some cases, destroys this potential. A psychic healer sees dis-ease as originating on the spiritual (etheric) level, progressing through the astral body, and showing itself in the mental body (the thoughts and memories that lead to our actions in life). Once the dis-ease "takes root" in these levels, physical symptoms appear. A practitioner of psychic healing seeks to clear blockages so that the process reverses itself. The psychic must then encourage an individual to resolve the original source of dis-ease.

There are many frauds in this field, so, as a consumer, you must be very careful about whom you choose to help you. Many scientists and nonscientists have criticized psychic healers, and you should be aware of these criticisms. *National Enquirer* (1975) and *Time* (1975) documented many (and indirectly *all*) psychic operations and cures as sleights of hands, animal matter used as diseased tissue, or roots that when liquified are the color of blood. However, there are still many cures that are unexplained and cannot be considered "great magic."

Psychics feel that they have an ability that is a basic human potential attainable by all people. They maintain that most people believe psi is something extraordinary or esoteric, whereas it is actually a natural experience that all of us have but few notice or recognize due to our beliefs about its extraordinary nature. Psychics offer some insights into their world that may be helpful in developing this so-called innate ability in each of us. Holistically oriented psychics assert that reality is seen from many perspectives and merges to form a "total" picture of an entity. For example, an inanimate object such as a table may seem lifeless, but to a psychic it is seen as a living conglomeration of energy given shape by the desires and thoughts of the table's owner. It is these desires and thoughts that reportedly direct the vital energy flow. Mental habits can shape psychic energies that lead to health or sickness. This simple formula of one choosing either a reality of wellness or a reality of illness is a fundamental tenet of psychic healing. However, this holistic account of psychic healing does not explain how the touch of a healer's hands can lead to a very quick cure, which is the way that one normally thinks of psychic healers.

It wasn't until 1927, when William McDougall moved to Duke University and hired J. B. and Louisa Rhine to study psi phenomena, that the scientific establishment took notice of paranormal activities. They were the first to study psychic phenomena in a laboratory setting. In 1933, the Rhines used Herbert Pearce, a famous psychic, to demonstrate that clairvoyance could be statistically validated. Upon hearing about these experiments, most of the scientific community exploded with counterclaims. Scientists said that the Rhines overlooked errors, that witnesses to psi acts were prejudiced, that there was no valid scientific experimentation, that lame theories were developed to account for the results, and that sensory cues were given to the ones being tested.

The Rhines developed the Zener cards, which contained five suits of stars, circles, crosses, squares, and wavy lines. Using these cards, they believe they statistically validated mental telepathy. Their experiments are important because they proved that psi activity was not locked into time, space, or the senses and because future experiments could be based upon the model discovered by them. Although no duplication of the Rhine experiments has been done, many other researchers have since that time validated *different* aspects of psi phenomena (G.N.M. Tyrrell, Dr. Soal, Graham and Anita Watkins, Delores Krieger, Bernard Grad, Thelma Moss, Gertrude Schmeidler, Michael Thalbourne, and Justa Smith, to name only a few). A significant number of other experiments under controlled conditions have been successful. Benjamin Wolman (1977), a distinguished scientist, and Edgar Mitchell (1974), the former astronaut, have demonstrated that information can be perceived without known channels of sensory information. Double-blind studies, however, have shown mixed results (Brier, Savits, and Schmeidler, 1974; Jacobson and Wiklund, 1976). Recent research at Duke has included experiments where the laying on of hands was found to improve plant growth. These experiments were double-blind and omitted the human factor. Researchers formed conclusions similar to the Rhines, suggesting that psychic healing is a valuable tool that modern medicine has overlooked (Grad, 1965; Smith, 1972).

Norman Shealy (1975), director of the Pain and Health Rehabilitation Center, and Delores Krieger (1979), a Ph.D. and a nurse practitioner, have also conducted tests. Shealy found that "intuitive diagnoses" (or using psychic healers for diagnoses) were 80 percent correct. Krieger teaches laying on of hands, or "therapeutic touch," to nurses at New York University, and although she has found no physiological explanation for it, she discovered that it worked on her subjects with a variety of disorders.

Dr. Thelma Moss, who is a leader of the movement that instituted a new law for both physicians and psychics to practice in California hospitals, suggests that those who wish to try psychic healing remain skeptical until they are convinced. She states that while many of us think of psychic healing as an instantaneous process, only one in ten thousand are healed the first time. In other words, psychic healing can be a long, slow process. Moss has used Kirlian photography to trace the energy fields long thought to exist by psychics and to show that energy can be transferred from one person to another.

These few studies exemplify psi's healing nature. We cannot report on all of the research done in psychic areas because volumes have been written both affirming and criticizing it. Consumers will have to be the final judges of psi's healing potentials. Experts do not believe that consumers should accept psi beyond any doubt. On the other hand, they point out, most individuals are aware of "unexplainable" events and acts that do occur. They recommend "a questioning attitude" to enable consumers to examine every possibility before deciding in favor of paranormal activity.

Alex Tanous, a noted psychic and teacher, says, "Learning to be psychic involves, at its core, learning to operate on the simplest levels, learning to accept the first images and impressions that flood your mind, instead of delving deeper" (1970). He explains that the major barriers preventing one from mastering psi skills are the temptation to go deeper with a thought, trying to pin down a thought and not waiting for "a feeling of certainty." With this information in mind, try the following exercises, which we have concocted from our research, making use of both your psi abilities and natural healing abilities.

Psi Healing Exercises

1. Relax in a quiet place. Breathe freely and deeply. Visualize (construct a scene in your mind in detail of) your body as whole and integrated. Imagine each part relying upon the other. Locate the area that is diseased and reconstruct it and its functions. Remember to trust the first impressions that cross your mind.

2. Relax and concentrate on one of these questions: What do I do to heal myself? What is causing my dis-ease? Note the symbolic images that pop into your head. Pay close attention to thoughts and phrases, for they may provide clues to the possible meaning of symbolic pictures.

3. Sit quietly and breathe deeply until you count to twenty. Exchange places with your dis-ease. Give it life, question it, ask why it came, ask what it needs in order to leave. You may want to write down your "conversation."

There are a number of "how to get ESP" books on the market. Although many of them do not specifically deal with healing, you should be able to adapt some of the exercises into healing activities.

In order more fully to comprehend psychic healing, it would be best if we had some general theory upon which to base it. It may not be difficult to accept the fact that our scientific theories are much too limited to explain this phenomenon. However, there are theories that present a psychological profile of the "potential" psychic; theories in physics that explain the lack of space-time involvement; medical theories that explore healing "after the fact," and theories that combine one or two of the others to explain the characteristics of healing. Surprisingly, there are no social theories, with the exception of tribal anthropological studies.

Researchers of psi phenomena are aware of this. Krippner and Villoldo (1976) call for a multidimensional theory, which includes psychological, psychic, medical, and physical phenomena. They, however, also excluded the need for social theories concerned with psi. Within healing, social theory can perhaps provide some insight into shared world views of the healer and client, personal qualities of both, symbols common to both, why one chooses "unconventional" healers, and the ways in which the expectations of the healers and healees affect the process of healing.

Psychic healers are not true holistic practitioners. The majority do not place emphasis on client-practitioner construction of a health program to promote well-being outside of the healing setting. In general, they do not include relaxation, nutrition, or exercise measures to supplement psychic healing. Practitioners point out that since psychic healing is supplemental to standard medical procedures, they feel that these areas are encountered by healees through medicine. However, advice in pertinent regions that affect energy imbalance is usually given to clients.

We found that some psychics, like spiritual healers, work in groups. The consumer is more likely to receive instruction on holistic areas of concern if he or she receives aid from a group of healers. It was explained to us that groups of healers are donating their time for the expressed purpose of healing. Their energies are directed to the healing of spiritual, mental, and physical energy deficits of the individual.

For the most part psychics do not talk about their abilities to others. They report that since there are a large numbers of frauds among psychic healers, they prefer to remain anonymous. Consumers will find that many psychic healers are licensed health professionals, such as psychiatrists and psychotherapists, who make use of psychic abilities within their practice. In other words, most legitimate psychics have allied themselves with structured medicine in order to be able to incorporate intuitive processes into medical science. It is their belief that this type of merger can only benefit the consumer who wishes treatment of physical, spiritual, and mental factors relating to dis-ease.

Type of Healing

Psychic healing can be classified as a natural method of healing because of its basic reliance upon natural laws. These laws are centered around the balance of the life force, communication between the individual and the creative force, relationships between energy centers and dis-ease, and pursuit of expanded consciousness. Additionally, their healing techniques involve nothing other than the healer and healee.

Psychic practitioners consider their work supplementary to standard medical care. Some request that you sign a form stating that you have been under a physician's care and have complied with the physician's treatment before they will see a client. They are careful to emphasize that they do not prescribe drugs, that they do not "treat" disease, and that their psychic ability may not clear energy blockages related to dis-ease. Other practitioners may ask that you document for their records your visit with them. Many of these healers keep documented case studies and/or statements from past clients to show to prospective clients. They also like to possess documented proof to pass on to the scientific community if asked.

Not all psychic practitioners heal by reading auras or chakras. A large number of these healers employ laying on of hands, yet they are not associated with organized religious doctrines. Some practitioners may speak in terms of "clearing the channels," and "balancing in order to prevent dis-ease." In other words, psychic practitioners who do not label themselves as spiritualists point out that they follow a broader (yet similar) religious doctrine.

We have already mentioned that there are many frauds among psychics. Within psychic healing, one must be especially wary of mediumship used as a way of contacting dead spirits in order to solve problems responsible for dis-ease. Psychics report that long, lost relatives *could* provide healing resolutions of guilt and unresolved problems, but we cannot recommend mediumship as a healing avenue, since most mediums require a seance. We are not saying that *all* mediums are frauds or that *all* seances are fake. We found, however, that this is the easiest psi area in which one can be exploited. Fred Archer (1966) warns, "except in the case of mediums . . . qualification is taken for granted. In their case the fraudulent is often equated with the norm."

We have included some tips for detecting fraudulent mediums and psychic healers below.

Consumer Tips for Spotting Fraudulent Healers and Mediums

1. Do not be "awed" by any display of debris from the body, trumpets, voices, materializations, or other "hocus pocus."
2. Do not have a fixed idea of what a psychic healer will do prior to the healing session or who a medium will contact in a seance.
3. Do not discuss personal affairs with a psychic healer or a medium or his or her staff.
4. Do not be impressed by famous persons who materialize for a medium or by those who heal many persons day after day.
5. Take notes during or immediately after a healing session or seance.
6. Do not be afraid to tell a healer that he or she has not cured you or to tell a medium that he or she is wrong.

7. If you get suspicious, check the room for concoctions or tissues, or wires and microphones.

8. Be careful of "ringers" who pretend to be healed but are actually members of the staff who are "healed" regularly.

9. Ask to talk with previous clients (privately) before agreeing to pay or participating in a session. Look for a way of confirming the psychic practitioner to your own satisfaction.

10. Only frauds guarantee results.

Beware of "psychic" fairs where astrology, tarot cards, and palm reading take place. Likewise, such local psychics as "Madam Sarah" or "Sister Teresa" may also be frauds. A good tip here is to try and work with psychic healers who are respected by a physician and/or those who have documented proof of their abilities.

Healers indirectly teach their clients about energy centers and how centers may be employed to detect the onset of dis-ease. Previous experiencers of psychic healing report a greater awareness of persons around them. Many former clients also state that they learned how to relax and allow natural body energies to flow evenly throughout the body. The skill was "picked up" through the healing settings, not by specific instruction by the healer. Practitioners affirm that their method of releasing blockages is an inhibited human ability. They add that many of their previous clients are able to preserve health by making use of techniques employed by psychic healers.

We have not offered you more proof of psi activity in healing than currently exists. Psychic healing continues to be disputed. Now, there are many fields which have entered the scientific arena who wish to provide concrete verification of psi events. The public, according to psychics, is more open to psi activity and as a result of their interest, more information about psi phenomena will be processed. At this time, however, the way in which psychic healers cure remains a mystery.

Description of Healing Method

We were not surprised to learn that "bona fide" psychic healers are few and far between. Clinics such as the ARE Clinic in Phoenix or Poseidia Institute in Virginia offer consumers the best of both worlds: medical professionals, psychic healers, natural treatments, and dietary emphasis. Generally, there are three kinds of healers in this field: those who work alone, those who work with the medical establishment in clinics and hospitals, and those who work as a group without the medical profession. Before we go further, it must be emphasized that the personal qualities of your healer are important to you, your compliance with the practitioner's recommendations and to the success of the cure. Consequently, we recommend that you search for someone whom you can easily relate to, someone you respect and get along with, and someone who shares similar viewpoints.

Set up an appointment. At this time ask if previous medical records are needed, if you will need to get your physician's signature, or if some type of documentation is required for the files. Remember that a practitioner may not ask you any details about earlier diagnoses, but this is dependent upon each healer. However, it often helps validate or legitimate a healer in the eyes of a consumer before undergoing their treatment.

If your psychic is affiliated with a medical clinic, expect to have a complete examination. Legitimate psychics feel that medical treatment is complementary and, in many cases, necessary in addition to their treatment. It is a good idea to take any extensive tests made in the recent past by other physicians in order to avoid unnecessary replication. Treatment is combined medical and natural. That is, physicians implement scientific principles and psychics usually supplement their treatment with laying on of hands, touch, or concentration. Treatments also include restructuring of habits deemed detrimental to personal well-being. Medical clinics such as the ARE include meditation, spiritual seminars, nutrition, exercise, and other measures to cure dis-ease. Settings that involve only psychiatrists and/or psychotherapists do not often offer this type of detailed treatment program for treating dis-eases. However, they may include educational seminars on such topics as nutrition, exercise, relaxation, and other methods. These are not required of patients but are encouraged as a means of promoting well-being.

Individual healers most often heal in their home. These healers can be personal and can devote a great deal of their time to counseling their clients. Unfortunately, this is not how many psychics treat patients. Most often, individual healers exert very little time toward counseling and restructuring. These healers are, as a rule, also more expensive.

We did locate a few practitioners who took time to instruct their clientele about health maintenance through relaxation and exercise. Overall, counseling on a one-to-one basis is the primary concern of individual psychic healers. They report that they do not necessarily (unless specifically requested by the client) encompass the components of holism into their practice. Instead, they point out, it is crucial that the client be able to shift conscious focus so that bodily processes can resume command. It is rare that healing takes place during the first experience with an independent psychic healer. Most report that, although improvement is noticeable immediately, a "cure" usually takes at least six separate treatment sessions.

Psychic centers often contain a group of psychics working together. They are like an "ordinary doctor's office" in appearance since there is a waiting room, a healing room, and sometimes, though not always, a counseling room. When you are called in for treatment, you will be asked what is bothering you. If any details are needed, the practitioner will ask for them. As mentioned before, you may be treated in a number of ways, but primarily by individual counseling and some sort of "touch" therapy. Do not be surprised if there are three or four tables in one room and healing is taking place all around you. Although many psychic clinics employ licensed health professionals and are located in newer office buildings, other legitimate practitioners find themselves in much more crowded conditions in older office buildings or homes. Healing centers composed exclusively of psychics and individual practitioners cannot prescribe drugs.

We should also expound upon the fact that according to most psychics, a client's expectations are key factors in the success of psychic healing. Those who expect to be "cleared of obstructions" will accomplish that. Those who expect clearing, counseling, changing, and balancing are also supposed to receive what they want. It is crucial, then, to ask the practitioner for holistic treatment if that is what you desire. This type of healing, accordingly, can be as general or as specific as you wish to make it. Psychics cannot overstep an imaginary boundary if you do not want them to or allow them to do so. This is your responsibility. So, if you want to get to the "bottom" of a dis-ease, take the time and energy to do so. On the other hand, if you want to clear up a dis-ease "now," your healer can only temporarily remove symptoms by clearing energy channels.

Diseases Treated

Psychic healers have reportedly cured the following dis-eases: obesity, smoking habit, stress-related conditions, high blood pressure, gastritis, colitis, abdominal pains, arthritis, bursitis, neuritis, asthma, liver conditions, liver diseases, phlebitis, cataracts, cerebral palsy, circulation problems, tumors, abscesses, cysts, dermatitis, diabetes, hemorrhoids, gallstones, kidney stones and kidney disease, pyorrhea, hay fever, hypoglycemia and hyperglycemia, jaundice, sinus infections, paralysis, psoriasis, rheumatism, removal of scars, tuberculosis, varicose veins, anemia, bladder problems, prostate disease, cancer, emphysema, paralysis, epilepsy, pleurisy, influenza, vertigo, spasms, gout, goiter and slipped disks.

Duration of Treatment

As you may have already surmised, cooperation between physicians and psychics in treating the whole person takes comparatively longer than visiting a group of psychics or an individual healer. The medical-psychic program encompasses testing, instruction, and counseling as well as diagnosis and treatment. You can plan on one month to six months from start to finish. But, according to practitioners, the effects of combined efforts and treatments are felt immediately. One former patient who attended the combined model type of clinic said, "I felt better after my second visit, but it took much longer to change my diet and my life and I needed them to help me do it." Another said, "I had a laying-on-of-hands treatment on my first visit. In subsequent visits I learned relaxation techniques, and I was given exercises for my condition. I also attended nutrition classes."

Psychic centers without medical staff operate differently. Objectively, it seems less personal simply because so much is going on around you. We feel that much of the reason it seems so impersonal is because practicing psychics in healing centers can be prosecuted for "treating or healing." So, quite naturally, these centers operate in secret.

Within this type of setting practitioners may vary with each visit, much like gynecologists or general practitioners working in the same office. Most clients return in consecutive weeks to receive treatments. Service and duration of the treatment is half that of a clinic. However, there is no counseling about diet, exercise, or other preventive health measures.

Psychic healers who work alone are oftentimes more involved with the total health of their clients, though some are not. Those who are can also be advisors, confidants, and role models. The problem here is that many individual practitioners are not knowledgeable enough in holistic principles to make recommendations for total well-being. Unless a practitioner "picks up" something specific relating to your problem, exercise and dietary education are frequently excluded from psychic care. You must make certain that your healer can provide these most vital components of holism, otherwise, he or she is not a holistic psychic. The length of treatments is highly individualized. You could possibly have one treatment, one treatment per day for five days, one treatment per week for six weeks or three treatments per week for several months. It is best to discuss this with the practitioner after the first treatment has been given.

Cost Range

Clinics—Medical and Psychic Combination
Initial visit—free–$50
                   $250–$475 per week (room and board included)
Follow-up visit—free–$40
Testing—$165–$250
Counseling—included with fees
Seminars—included with fees or $15–$30 per class

Centers
Initial visit—free–$30
Follow-up visit—free–$30
Counseling—included with fees

Individual Healers
Initial visit—free–$25
Follow-up visit—free–$20
Counseling—free–$20

Personal Responsibilities

Perhaps the most important responsibility you have when working with a psychic healer is to yourself. Your willingness to expand and open yourself can "make or break" a psychic cure. Remember that healers using the holistic method are looking at reality from many different angles. They will ask that you try and do the same. Changing your perception, psychics argue, allows you the opportunity to gain a sense of self. A "sense of self" is needed to change the focus of your attention from "I" to "All." Accompanied by a willingness to heal yourself, an "all" consciousness (consideration, feeling, and equality) is the basis for preventing dis-ease and maintaining the life force. If you do not agree with these values, psychic healing may not work for you.

Interview previous clients who have made use of your practitioner. Find out what illnesses were treated, how long it took, the payment, and if he or she included diet and exercise as part of the therapy. Ask questions about the healer's reputation to determine if the practitioner is consistent with your conception of "a healer." However, do not be so skeptical that you come on like a district attorney! Satisfy yourself, to the best of your ability, that the healer is bona fide.

Psychic healers place healing responsibility upon the individual. Do not be afraid to ask a practitioner what would help maintain energy flow, although you may not wish to comply with his or her answer. Since it is a fact that most groups of psi healers and many individual practitioners do not integrate health preservation measures within their healing practices, consumers must add maintenance techniques to their life-style on their own. Psychic practice is designed to encourage growth and awareness of the individual aspects relating to dis-ease. Compliance with a healer's recommendations combined with a self-search for healing possibilities incorporates both client and practitioner as a team in the healing process. Be sure to express to the healer that you prefer holistic treatment if you feel it will best suit your needs.

Because of the "uncertainty" and "power" attributed to psychics, many consumers tend to assume that this realm of healing is a panacea for any and all dis-eases. Practitioners explain that one cannot live haphazardly and be continually "cleared" by psychics. For one thing, genuine concern for health is viewed as how well one takes responsibility for well-being. For another, many psychics will not see clients who continually disregard health.

Become aware of your dis-ease. Study up on it and read about others who have experienced the same problem. This will protect you from being overwhelmed or gullible about the dis-ease and a healer's ability to cure you. In addition, it will make you knowledgeable enough about the subject to enable you to begin healing by using what you discover, rather than relying upon others. The psychic healing exercises presented earlier will help initiate psi healing activity. They can unlock self-healing potential or balance bodily functions.

Finally, do not allow a medium to heal through a seance no matter what argument you are given. Find another healer.

Informational Organizations

Association for Documentation
and Enlightenment, Inc.
314 Arctic Crescent
Virginia Beach, VA 23451

The Nirvana Foundation for
Psychic Research
138 West Campbell Avenue
Campbell, CA 95008

Poseidia Institute, Centers for
Interdisciplinary Research
PO Box 180
Virginia Beach, VA 23458

Association for Research
and Enlightenment
PO Box 595
Virginia Beach, VA 23451

Florida Society for Psychical Research, Inc.
4312 46th Avenue South
St. Petersburg, FL 33711

Consistencies

1. Deficits in energy centers, as in acupuncture, cause manifestation of dis-ease on any level. Psychics place the responsibility for healing on the consumer. A practitioner can only assist by clearing or reducing energy blockages.

2. As with most other methods, psychic healers work with intangible "energies," "centers," "blockages," and "distributions." This aspect of holistic theory is clearly expressed by psychics.

3. The expense of psychic healing sessions is often negotiable. The average donation is $10 to $20 for each session. Psychics, then, are less expensive than more conventional healers.

4. Viewpoints of the world should be in close conjunction with the healer chosen. This contributes to a strong foundation in order for healing to be completed.

5. The laying on of hands or therapeutic touch is currently being utilized and taught in nursing programs. The basics of psi healing are being employed by legitimate health professionals in conjunction with allopathic medicine and modern science. The clinical techniques of nutritional and emotional counseling are also used by nurse practitioners. Furthermore, Arthur Hastings recommends the techniques of intuitive diagnosis used by psychic healers as an integral part of modern medicine. Finally, Thelma Moss has been instrumental in proving the existence of the electromagnetic energies that make up the psychic realm. Some very important scientists see psychic healing as a potential contributor to the future of medicine.

Inconsistencies

1. This method is more controversal than the other methods presented in this book. The reason is that the most important inconsistency within psychic healing is that these healers do not directly treat the mind and body because their focus is centered on the spirit. The majority do not give recommendations for dietary changes or exercise. Rather than being multidimensional, they only rely upon one dimension.

2. Many practitioners in this field say that they require the patient to first engage the services of orthodox physicians. Yet many are known to give consultations and healing through the mail. Additionally, how could one validate the prerequisite unless a massive envelope containing all the tests is sent?

3. During our research we found only sparse theories that attempted to explain psi functions. The most impressive was born in quantum physics. It is odd that no one within psi science has formed a more thorough theoretical explanation of this phenomena.

4. Scientists may balk if we do not include the fact that the research into psi is biased. However, we feel that anyone researching any field is doing so because he or she wants to expand that field. The experiments within psi science controlled the variables as well as a chemist would in what scientists refer to as double-blind experiments. The charge of sensory cues is ridiculous because of this reason. However, you need to be aware of this controversy before becoming a patient of a psychic healer.

5. Unfortunately, psi areas are practiced by many who are not psychics. Consequently, there are many fraudulent healers in this field.

Sources to Read

Agee, Doris. *Edgar Cayce on E.S.P.* New York: Hawthorn Books, 1969.

Angoff, Allan. *Eileen Garret and the World Beyond the Senses.* New York: William Morrow, 1974.

Archer, Fred. *Crime and the Psychic World.* New York: William Morrow, 1969.

——. *Exploring the Psychic World.* New York: William Morrow, 1966.

Atkinson, William W. *Psychic Healing.* London: Yoga Publishing, 1970.

Bach, Marcus. *The Power of Perception.* Garden City, NY: Doubleday, 1965.

Bagnall, Oscar. *Origin and Properties of the Human Aura.* New York: Weiser, 1970.

Bailey, Alice A. *Esoteric Healing.* London and New York: Lucis Publishing Co., 1953.

Bauman, Edward, et al. *The Holistic Health Handbook.* Berkeley, CA: And/Or Press, 1978.

Bohm, D. J. "A Suggested Interpretation of the Quantum Theory in Terms of Hidden Variables, I and II," *Physical Review,* 85, 1952, pp. 166 to 179, 180 to 193.

Brier, Robert; Savits, B.; and **Schmeidler, G.** "Experimental Tests of Silva Mind Control Graduates," in *Research in Parapsychology,* ed. William Roll et al. Metuchen, NJ: Scarecrow Press, 1974.

Burr, H. S. *The Fields of Life.* New York: Ballantine, 1973.

Cayce, Hugh Lynn. *Venture Inward.* New York: Harper and Row, 1964.

Cohen, David. *E.S.P.: The Search Beyond the Senses.* New York: Harcourt Brace Jovanovich, 1973.

DeLong Miller, Roberta. *Psychic Massage.* New York: Harper and Row, 1974.

Dimensions of Healing. Los Altos, CA: Academy of Parapsychology and Medicine, 1972.

Dooley, A. *Every Wall a Door: Exploring Psychic Surgery and Healing.* London: Abelard Schuman, 1972.

Ebon, Martin. *Prophecy in Our Time.* New York: New American Library, 1968.

————. *The Psychic Reader.* New York: World Publishing Company, 1969.

————. *They Knew the Unknown.* New York: World Publishing Company, 1971.

Ebon, Martin, ed. *The Psychic Scene.* New York: Signet, 1974.

Edwards, Harry. *The Healing Intelligence.* New York: Hawthorn Books, 1974.

Fishbein, N. *Fads and Quakery in Healing.* New York: Covci and Freide, 1932.

Godwin, Hohn. *Occult America.* Garden City, NY: Doubleday, 1972.

Grad, Bernard. "Some Biological Effects of the 'Laying-on-of-Hands:' A Review of Experiments with Animals and Plants," *Journal of the American Society for Psychical Research* 59, no. 2 (April 1965), pp. 95–126.

Hastings, Arthur; Fadiman, James; Gordon, James, eds. *Health for the Whole Person.* Boulder, CO: Westview, 1981.

Haynes, Reneè. *The Hidden Springs: An Enquiry into Extra Sensory Perception.* Boston: Little, Brown, 1973.

Heisenberg, W. *Physics and Beyond.* New York: Harper and Row, 1972.

Herbert, B. "Theory and Practice of Psychic Healing," *Parapsychology Review,* November–December, 1975, pp. 22–23.

Holms, Campbell A. *The Facts of Psychic Science.* New Hyde Park, NY: University Books, 1969.

Hudson, Thomas J. *The Law of Psychic Phenomena.* New York: Weiser, 1968.

Jacobson, N., and **Wiklund, N.** "Investigation of Claims of Diagnosing by Means of E.S.P.," in *Research in Parapsychology,* William Roll et al. Metuchen, NJ: Scarecrow Press, 1976.

Kaslof, Leslie J. *Wholistic Dimensions in Healing.* Garden City, NY: Doubleday, 1978.

Kilner, Walter J. *The Human Aura.* New York: Weiser, 1973.

Kinnear, W., ed. *Thought as Energy.* Los Angeles: Science of Mind, 1975.

Klein, Aaron E. *Beyond Time and Matter: A Sensory Look at ESP.* Garden City, NY: Doubleday, 1973.

Krieger, Delores. *The Therapeutic Touch: How to Use Your Hands to Help or to Heal.* Englewood Cliffs, NJ: Prentice-Hall, 1979.

Krieger, Delores; Peper, E.; and **Ancoli, S.** "Therapeutic Touch: Searching for Evidence of Physiologic Change," *American Journal of Nursing* 4 (April 1979): 784–787.

Krippner, Stanley, and **Rubin, D.,** eds. *The Energies of Consciousness.* New York: Gordon and Breach, 1975.

Krippner, Stanley, and **Villoldo, A.** *The Realms of Healing.* Millbrae, CA: Celestial Arts, 1976.

Kruger, Helen. *Other Healers Other Cures.* New York: Bobbs Merrill, 1974.

Le Shan, Lawrence. *The Medium, The Mystic and The Physicist.* New York: Ballantine, 1975.

McCreery, Charles. *Psychic Phenomena and the Physical World.* New York: Ballantine, 1973.

Mishlove, Jeffery. *Roots of Consciousness—Psychic Liberation through History, Science and Experience.* New York: Random House, 1975.

Mitchell, Edgar D., et al., eds. *Psychic Exploration.* New York: Putnam's, 1974.

Moss, Thelma, Ph.D. *The Body Electric: A Personal Journey into the Mysteries of Parapsychological Research, Bioenergy and Kirlian Photography.* Los Angeles, CA: J. P. Tarcher, 1979.

Nash, J. C. "Medical Parapsychology," *Parapsychology Review.* January–February 1972, pp. 13–18.

Ostrander, Sheila, and **Schroeder, L.** *Handbook of Psi Discoveries.* New York: Putnam's, 1974.

Porter, Jean. *Psychic Development.* New York: Random House, 1974.

Pratt, G. J. *Parapsychology: An Insider's View of E.S.P.* Garden City, NY: Doubleday, 1964.

Rhine, J. B. *Extrasensory Perception.* Boston: Bruce Humphries, 1964.

——. *New World of the Mind.* New York: William Morrow, 1953.

——. *The Reach of the Mind.* New York: William Sloane Associates, 1960.

Rhine, J. B., and **Brier, R.,** eds. *Parapsychology Today.* New York: The Citadel Press, 1968.

Rhine, Louisa E. *Mind over Matter.* New York: Macmillan, 1970.

Roberts, Jane. *The Seth Series.* Englewood Cliffs, NJ: Prentice-Hall, 1966–81.

Schmeidler, Gertrude, and **McConnell, R.** *E.S.P. and Personality Patterns.* New Haven, CT: Yale University Press, 1958.

Shealy, Norman C., with **Freese, A. S.** *Occult Medicine Can Save Your Life: A Modern Doctor Looks at Unconventional Healing.* New York: Dial, 1975.

Sherman, Harold. *Wonder Healers of the Philippines.* Santa Monica, CA: De Vorss, 1967.

——. *Your Mysterious Powers of E.S.P.* New York: World Publishing, 1969.

——. *Your Power to Heal.* Greenwich, CT: Fawcett, 1972.

Smith, Eleanor T. *Psychic People.* New York: William Morrow, 1968.

Smith, Grover, ed. *The Letters of Aldous Huxley.* New York: Harper and Row, 1969.

Smith, Sister M. J. "Paranormal Effects on Enzyme Activity through Laying-on-of-Hands," *Human Dimensions I,* Spring 1972, pp. 15–19.

Spraggett, Allen. *The Unexplained.* New York: New American Library, 1967.

Spraggett, Allen, and **Rauscher, W. V.** *The Psychic Mafia.* New York: Harper and Row, 1975.

Steiner, Lee. *Psychic Healing for Psychological Problems.* Englewood Cliffs, NJ: Prentice-Hall, 1967.

Stevenson, Ian. "Healing: A Doctor in Search of a Miracle," *Journal of the American Society for Psychical Research,* 70, 1976, pp. 101–108.

Sturzaker, James. *Twelve Rays.* New York: Weiser, 1976.

Tanous, Alex, with **Ardman, H.** *Beyond Coincidence: One Man's Experiences with Psychic Phenomena.* Garden City, NY: Doubleday, 1970.

Valentine, Thomas. *Psychic Surgery.* New York: Pocket Books, 1975.

Van Vliet, Cornelius J. *Varieties of Healing Experience.* Los Altos, CA: Academy of Parapsychology and Medicine, 1973.

Vaughn, Alan. "Investigation of Silva Mind Control Claims," in *Research in Parapsychology,* ed. William Roll et al. Metuchen, NJ: Scarecrow Press, 1974.

————. *Patterns of Prophecy.* New York: Hawthorn Books, 1974.

Vaughn, Frances. *Awakening Intuition.* New York: Doubleday, 1979.

Walker, E. H. "Consciousness as a Hidden Variable," *Physics Today,* 1971, pp. 24–39.

Walker, Evan H. "Science/Consciousness/Religion," in W. Kinner, ed., *Thought as Energy.* Los Angeles: Science of Mind, 1975.

Watts, Alan. *Cloud-Hidden, Whereabouts Unknown.* New York: Pantheon, 1961.

Weil, Andrew. *The Natural Mind.* Boston: Houghton Mifflin, 1972.

White, George, M.D. *Finer Forces of Nature in Diagnosis and Therapy.* Mokelumme Hill, CA: Health Research, 1969.

White, John, ed. *Psychic Exploration.* New York: Putnam's, 1974.

Wolman, Benjamin. *Handbook of Parapsychology.* New York: Van Nostrand Reinhold, 1977.

10

NATIVE AMERICAN HEALING

Definition

When the exodus from Europe to the New World occurred, the settlers, many sick from the long voyage, turned to Native Americans for their expertise in healing and preventing dis-ease through the use of North American herbs and foods. European healers had employed "bleeding" as a technique for healing. When the shaman's medicine (consisting of healing ceremonies and herbs) was compared with the apparent barbarism of "bleeding," Native American healers gained the friendship and patronage of the early settlers. Virgil Vogel put it another way, "The Shaman was often successful, not only in the treatment of Indians, but also whites. Most writers have attributed this success at least in part to psychological factors not recognized in earlier times but given much attention today" (Vogel, 1970).

Vogel, who has written an excellent account of Native American relations with the settlers, points out that the settlers wrote home describing the American Indians as extremely clean. They bathed every day, were not deformed, and remained in excellent physical condition. Also, they had clean white teeth and kept neatly swept huts and villages. Contrastingly, the settlers seldom bathed, practiced very few "cleanliness habits," and were continually sick.

Ironically, the ceremonies that were performed by the Indians to accompany herbs and other methods were responsible for the racial bias by the settlers. They considered the rituals savagery, unaware that the Native American was cognizant of a far greater interrelationship between man, nature, the universe, and the psyche. Instead, it was the Indian mode of dress, symbolic ritual, and simplistic living style that earned them the title of "primitive."

Generalizations about Indian culture and civilization run the risk of stereotyping Native Americans and increasing prejudice against them. One must be careful to avoid viewing Indians as one tribe or culture. Each tribe is actually its own nation with its own distinctive language and beliefs. The most common elements shared by these tribes are the importance of religion and a natural view of the world, along with a belief in the power of people to heal themselves. Native Americans believe that man and the universe are interdependent. In order to maintain harmony and wholeness, man acknowledges and works with all of the energies in nature, some of which may not be visible.

Indians believe that body centers must remain free from contention so that energy remains free flowing. In order to replenish the vital force when negative energies have accumulated, one is taught to balance one's desires and interests with environmental forces. Man is never viewed as separate from the earth but as an integral part of it. Native Americans, then, incorporate holism into their healing philosophy.

The basis of Native American medicine stems from the belief in the coexistence of man and nature. The earth is viewed as a living organism. Mother Earth can teach one how to give and take from her inhabitants without destroying the fruits of her breast. Indian societies learned from observance of Mother Nature to make use of natural laws including energy forces, herbs, and mental strategies. Physical objects that are a part of nature such as rocks, feathers, and colored sands are living, contain energy, and have spiritual sides. They can, therefore, be used in healing. According to most Indian religions, the Great Spirit guides the medicine man (or woman) because he or she lives in accordance with these natural laws of respect for Mother Earth and her inhabitants. They believe that if honor is not paid to Mother Nature, disease, famine, poverty, and societal conflict can befall an individual and the tribe.

Native American ceremonies are celebratory prayers that concretely express man's interrelationship to the natural world. They also believe that these rituals dissipate and/or create energy needed to sustain Mother Earth, her inhabitants, and the entire universe. Rolling Thunder, perhaps the most famous Native American healer of today, states that we can learn to control our energies just as we learn to walk. But, the Great Spirit and Mother Earth must be allowed to make their presence known within the individual first. Rolling Thunder has faith that, according to ancient Indian prophecy, creative spiritual endeavor will change both the white man's perception of the Indian and the white man's destruction of nature. In his words, "The spirit is returning to the Indians and is extending to young people across the country. Many of them are becoming spiritual warriors. That doesn't mean they are going to make war. Being a spiritual warrior means becoming a complete person. It means having consideration for other people, and in finding spirituality through truth and beauty" (Krippner and Villoldo, 1976, p. 69).*

The healing ceremony is only one of many rituals in Native American society. These rituals contain music, dance, song, prayer, and social interaction and depict man's relationship to the whole. Spiritual celebration reiterates man's connection with self, others, nature, and the cosmos. Ceremonial prayers are offered as greetings, sacrifices, respect, and pleasure, all envoking harmony with the environment.

Once again, as in other holistic modalities, we encounter the vital force as an healing energy. It is portrayed in most aspects of Indian ritual and life. Herbs release their energy when grown and prepared in a specific manner; Mother Earth creates and releases energy when prayers and dances are performed correctly; the healee receives healing energies when he or she allows energy to flow smoothly and conquers dis-ease in a personal manner.

Native Americans also believe that energy flows through energy centers like chakras. Ceremonial dances and songs sustain the energy flow. This is one reason why the healing dance is performed barefooted. Electromagnetic energy from the earth is supposed to flow up through the feet of the dancer and then is stored for transference to the healee. Additionally, bare feet enable the shaman to expel negative energy back to Mother Earth. The life force is released to the healee at the climax of the healing ritual after the shaman has sufficiently gathered the "force," cleansed the patient, and prepared him or her for the reception of healing power.

Another belief encompassed in Native American healing is the idea of cyclical processes that are symbolized by the round formation of dances, drums, and ceremonies for several types of activities: planting, harvesting, and the change of seasons, birth, hunting, peace, and social

*Reprinted courtesy Celestial Arts Publishing Co., Millbrae, California.

conflict among others. The cosmic universe is circular, just as rebirths and deaths of human beings. These rituals are continual reaffirmations of ideals which state that where there is an end, there is a beginning; where there is darkness, there is light; or where there is winter, there will be spring. The cyclical motion of life, then, is a never-ending process that comes full circle when health is sought in the midst of dis-ease. Not only do these beliefs provide hope, they also inculcate the belief that Mother Nature maintains a dynamic balance between all the elements of the universe.

With the use of drums, herbs, sweats, chants, and dances a "healing mood" is created by the shaman. The language of the healing chant is complicated. Chants, "a way," "a sing," and songs within healing ceremonies are stories or myths about heroes and heroines that go through struggles in the supernatural realm to learn their cures, over-whelm the dis-ease, bring the cure back to the healee and tribe, and are healed. Greek myths coincide with stories performed by song and dance in Native American culture. Dancers perform specific steps to enact the plot of a story as a part of all rituals. The drumbeat provides the "regularity" of life and the heartbeat as it enhances the eradication of dis-ease during a healing ceremony.

Remedies are chosen according to the "doctrine of signatures," or the homoeopathic theory that like cures like. To the Indian healer the liverleaf is used to treat liver ailments because the leaves of the plant resemble the liver (An interesting sideline was noted in a children's book on Indian crafts that also relates to the doctrine of signatures. The author states that Native Americans did not eat much sugar because they observed the branches of maple trees swaying in the wind. This was interpreted as meaning those who ate sugar would likely get dizzy [Salomon, 1928]). The "like cures like" theory of choosing herbs is not always used. Supernatural visions and trial and error experimentation also provide Native Americans with plants that cure their dis-eases. You might be thinking that the Native American "system" of choosing plant life to cure is backward. But, many holistic medical theories are also based upon observance of natural laws and native flora.

Native American healers are as specialized as modern healers. Remember that chants and dances are individual or clan possessions. One clan may know the prayers and dances to evoke success upon a married couple, whereas another clan may possess chants and dances for blessing a new home. Similarly, one practitioner may have learned the ritual for healing animal wounds, but another would have to be summoned to perform the healing ceremony to treat a difficult preg-nancy.

Native American healers also demonstrate a knowledge of purifi-cation by water and/or steam. Massage and manipulation are frequently used in treatment, as is simple surgery. To ensure that energy flows smoothly, massage and manipulation with natural substances are put to use as exercise. These are commonly employed in combination with forms of hydrotherapy. Steam baths were invented by Native Americans to rid the body of poisons through sweats and have evolved into purification rituals in Native American healing.

Today, many problems exist between Indian and white Americans that prevent most consumers from making use of Indian healing measures. Some of these conflicts are focused on the very basic symbolic representations of the two cultures. Medical acknowledgment of Native American contributions to the healing sciences is one area that seems to be making progress for both cultures. The U.S. Indian Health Service and tribal shamans are now exchanging practitioners in hopes of bridging the gap between traditional and nontraditional healing. In the early 1970s the Department of Health, Education and Welfare funded a project to train Navaho shamans, since they could more effectively deal with some disorders that more conventional physicians did not understand and which were prevalent in the Indian nations.

In many Indian nations today there are major conflicts between members of the tribal council who advocate and work with the Bureau of Indian Affairs and the Native Americans that advocate traditional leadership. Because of these contentions many stereotypes still exist. Due to the competitive hostility between the BIA, younger tribal leaders, and traditional leaders, we do not recommend that consumers contact a Native American healer by way of the BIA. The U.S. Indian Health Service seems to be the simplest means of contacting health clans, if there are any in your area. They will take your name and pass it on to healers, although this is still not a guarantee that one will be reached.

Another contingency that strains interchange between our two cultures is a core belief among Native Americans: Mother Earth, the central spirit of creation, allows all people to live upon her. In return, she asks, according to Native American cultures, that we take care of her. Water and air pollution and the mining of uranium for nuclear power plants on reservation lands threaten the very roots of Indian survival. According to Indian beliefs, water pollution destroys fishing, a major food source, air pollution destroys crop production, manufacturing processes destroy desert water tables; and mining of reservation lands destroys Native American health as well as their land and religion. And, many Indians say they have nothing else. Native Americans point out that current energy problems will not be "cured" by destroying yet another culture. Native Americans from all regions are currently struggling with the government over these issues.

In some ways white Americans are learning from Native Americans, for the American Indian is widely portrayed as a symbol of ecology. And, justly so. They are America's cultural symbols of the spiritual, mental, emotional, and physical link to Mother Earth. This person is often portrayed in conservation and solar energy public service announcements. Until recently, the value of the Indian nations to medicine, pharmacology, culture, and art has largely been obscured. After completing our research, we began to believe that understanding the culture that maintained this land long before most of us arrived here should be as important to our learning as understanding the conflicts that led us to America. Native Americans were among the first holistic healers, incorporating spirit, mind, and body into a philosophy of healing that relied upon the power of individuals to heal themselves. Ritualistic healing ceremonies, backed by years of apprenticeship, emphasized symbolic cures and prevention of dis-ease rather than merely the physical components of illness. Using a variety of techniques ranging from herbs to minor surgery and hydrotherapy, the shaman was a combination spiritual leader and physician. Currently, there is a resurgence of Native American healers at a time when the spiritual and mental dimensions of healing are just being reviewed by modern medicine.

Type of Healing Method

Donald Sandner (1978), speaking about Navaho shamans, said that they "understand intuitively that there are at least two kinds of healing: scientific healing based on anatomy and physiology, and symbolic healing that focuses on the cultural being and the symbolic universe that provides human consciousness.* Native American healers are aware, then, that more than one method may be needed to cure a specific dis-ease. They will persuade one to go to a clinic or hospital if the medicine required is beyond the scope of their knowledge and/or expertise.

Measures taken in healing involve the forces of unity. That is, energies from Mother Nature's gifts perpetuate the healing setting. Herbs, water therapies, fasting, prayers, touch, and symbolic healing tools combine forces to initiate the healing state within the healee. The healer's "power" is used to replace the lack of "power" in the one who is ill.

The chant, being an integral part of Indian society, needs to be

*From "Navaho Medicine" by Donald F. Sandner, *Human Nature*, July 1978. Copyright © 1978 by Human Nature, Inc. Reprinted by permission of the publisher.

explained before one seeks help from a Native American healer. A chant encompasses the healee's struggles, searching, and control over dis-ease. Through dance, plot, remedies, rhythm, beat, symbols, and ritual the shaman creates a picture that expresses harmony, rebirth, vitality, and will to live. Furthermore, all emotions such as love, confusion, and wellness are expressed in chants. The shaman never doubts the power of ritual and prayer to heal.

The healing process usually contains five basic stages: purification, evocation, identification, transformation, and release. Each plays a crucial part in effecting cures. More than one shaman usually participates in the ritual. Payment, however, is made to the one who performs the chant and is the leader of the healing ceremony.

Ceremonies work because the *patient* completes the healing process. The shaman attends, organizes, symbolizes, re-creates, and nourishes the healing process. The healee is the total focus of friends and family as well as the healers. All these people participate in chants and prayers. After the healing ritual has been finished, an all-night sing, complete with dance, song, and food, is planned for the healee. Their individual attentions are concentrated upon the celebration of *wellbeing*. After this, one would be embarrassed by remaining ill.

The healing process of chanting usually takes four days and nights. Because of its great importance in the Native American healing ceremony, we have roughly condensed the chant's purpose in the box below.

Native American Healing Chant

DAY	CHANT THEME
1	Cleansing and blessings by the Great Spirit.
2	God's battles to rid the body of disease.
3	Healee's battle with and resolution of the dis-ease.
4	Restoration of beauty and happiness of the body as a whole.

As you can see, the healing ceremony includes most of the traits of holism. The body is cleansed and purified. Native Americans believe that the medicinal energies of herb teas combine with electromagnetic energy from Mother Earth to stimulate the body centers of the healee. Linguistic symbols provide the "setting" and "plot" in which healing occurs. The patient is the central character who *experiences* both internal and external healing. Shamans instill ideal spiritual, mental, and physical states that are, thereby, "constructed" simultaneously by the healer and healee. These new "constructions" of health are then shared with the community so that they, too, can make use of the insights gained by the experience. Additionally, one can observe how the community becomes a social support system for the healee, thereby reinforcing the experience.

It is easy to conclude that Native American healing measures are natural because their medical "science" is based upon the method of natural observations. Symbols, celebrations, and techniques are chosen because of connections that are believed to exist. Indian healing measures are complicated due to the fact that thousands of years of observation have been passed down from healer to healer. These natural processes are believed to re-create healing energy in all realms of disease: spiritual, mental, and physical. Native Americans have grounded their lives in a harmonious superstructure that supports and enhances all life. They assume that Mother Earth, the symbol of creation, perpetuates the vital force in order for life on earth to continue. There are relatively few Native American physicians who have attended orthodox medical establishments; the number is so small that they are unable to take care of the demands placed upon them. For these practitioners, traditional Native American practices can ease their load. Cooperation between symbolic healers and modern Western healing techniques is a contemporary trend. As modern physicians learn of the significance of this type of healing modality, we add to our own storehouse of knowledge.

Description of Healing Method

In earlier days, Anglo and Native American lived in close proximity. Now, however, it is much harder for white Americans to be treated by Indian healers. Since Native Americans have been isolated in reserved areas, one must consider the expense it would take to reach a healer unless one lives near a reservation or knows the nearby location of a particular practitioner. Once there, one must find the medicine society or clan to have the dis-ease treated. Obtaining permission may take quite a while. Unfortunately, it's an involved process but not something that cannot be overcome if money and time are available to the healee.

Practitioners that make use of laying on of hands hold their hands over a body to locate "cold spots" within the patient. These are the areas that need treatment. Other healers employ "shaking hands" in the same manner with the exception being that the healer points to the parts that are "out of balance." Aura reading, crystal balls, or night stars are other diagnostic tools that may lead a practitioner to the source of dis-ease (Sandner, 1978;* Waters, 1963).

Some Native Americans believe that energy can also be controlled by healing crystals. It is said that crystals must be taken in natural form from the earth and given as a gift to the shaman. The "electromagnetic energy" contained within the crystals turns them hot or cold when they are brought into contact with the human aura. When passed over a dis-eased body, they believe that a crystal draws out "bad energies," allowing the body "a breather," so to speak, to enable it to "rediscover" the correct balance, which was previously inhibited.

Dream therapy (see Chapter 13) is also used by Indians. The literature states that both Iroquois and Cherokee healers have excelled in using dream analysis as a healing tool (Krippner and Villoldo, 1976; Otto and Knight, 1979; Vogel, 1970). Most practitioners (in these tribes) will ask about dreams that occurred immediately after the onset of dis-ease. The psyche usually tells one, according to dream healers, what is wrong before dis-ease manifests itself on the physical level. Often healers believe that they are able to pinpoint energy channels that are clogged. The practitioner, by applying his or her knowledge of the universe and the healee, is able to create a new dream sequence to accompany the other practices in healing.

Once you have made contact with a healer, he or she will determine the nature of your dis-ease. This does not mean that a practitioner desires the diagnosis of a previous healer. He or she just wants the symptoms. Let the healer ask the questions. Most healers do not perform a general physical examination except when only one healer is involved in the examination. Your fee will be paid to the healer you choose. Ordinarily, the practitioner will pay any assistants (such as attendants, drummers, or dancers) who participate in the ceremony. Fees are negotiable or left for bartering.

After the diagnosis is made, a fee is discussed (see "Cost Range"), and a time and date are set for the healing ceremony. Treatment usually begins on the day diagnosis is made, but occasionally other practitioners from another clan may be needed and time is required for their arrival. A ceremony for healing will last from four to seven days, and your family may be allowed to observe and participate during the rites.

Treatment begins with cleansing and purifying of the healee. A specially prepared "medicine lodge" will be used for these purposes. Herbal emetics and teas cleanse and nourish the body. A fire is built

---

*Adapted from "Navaho Medicine" by Donald F. Sandner, Human Nature, July 1978. Copyright © 1978 by Human Nature, Inc. Reprinted by permission of the publisher.

inside the lodge in which rocks are heated. Sage and cedar are employed as sweating herbals. Water is splashed on the rocks to produce steam. The combination of emetics, teas, and steam eliminates the body poisons. Fasting the length of the ceremony further assures that no toxins enter the body after it has been purified. This process takes from thirty minutes to an hour and a half, depending upon the body's condition.

After cleansing has taken place, you are moved to another dwelling. It is here that the healing ceremony will be performed. Herbal oils are applied to your purified body. Massage and manipulation are used to correct posture, loosen muscles, and provide exercise. This is a very soothing procedure. Your body is pampered, nourished, and blessed for the upcoming battle with dis-ease. This accomplished, you are left to rest. Although you are not allowed to eat solid foods, an herbal remedy or broth is left to drink.

No doubt, some of these practices will seem rugged. However, the "rawness" of it does not mean that this method does not work. Because of this, we have explicitly explained some of the symbolism and meaning integrated into the Native American healing ceremony. Indian culture is created by acknowledging the coexistence of body, mind, spirit, and universe, which reflects a multidimensional view. Their ceremonies and day-to-day life are supposed to enact this belief. Prayer songs include their search for renewed harmony among themselves, others, and the world. Consequently, ceremonies are a regular part of Indian society. It is their belief that their prayers, songs, chants, dances, and rituals can and do effect change in the universe that forms the foundation for healing.

Diseases Treated

Native Americans feel that dis-ease is caused by disharmony in the individual in relation to the tribe and the world around him or her. For this reason, dis-ease is viewed as manifestation of dis-harmony and is treated by re-creating harmony in the body centers. Serious dis-ease and internal problems are treated by physicians who may or may not be Native American. The ailments treated by Indians include burns, boils, pregnancy, bursitis, abscesses, crusty eyes, calluses, arthritis, rheumatism, phlegm, spinal disorders, chorea, diabetes, scurvy, circulation problems, constipation, cysts, tumors, earaches, depression, dermatitis, diarrhea, eye problems, respiratory ailments, scalds, fevers, slipped disks, eczema, dislocations, frostbite, fractures, sprains, strains, goiter, hemorrhoids, worms, hypertension, gastritis, menstrual problems, phlebitis, pleurisy, poisonous bites and itches, and mental imbalances.

Duration of Treatment

The length of time that is required to treat dis-ease varies from one healer to another. In general, four to fourteen days are needed for total treatment. Remember, these practitioners serve dual community functions: healers and priests. The double nature of their role, therefore, appears in the healing ceremony. Ordinarily, a minimum of four days is required to encompass the four major directions of healing and obtain their powers and blessings for healing. Ceremonies to re-create general harmony between the healee and his or her self, community, environment, and body continue for four to six days. This healing rite envokes "all the powers that be" to help one maintain health as well as disperse all dis-harmony.

For more complicated diseases, treatment is lengthened. For example, one may suffer from many mental and physical symptoms that must be drawn away from the healee. One may have oozing boils, itchy skin, and overweightness as physical symptoms, accompanied by a snappish attitude, depression, and ineffectiveness and lack of productivity at work. Many Native American healers, like homoeopaths, work on pairs of symptoms, effecting harmony in one before treating the next. The aforementioned healee would be relieved of boils and inactivity first and foremost and obesity and snappish attitude last. Light diet and herbal remedies provide "follow-up" practices. These precautions are usually taken for four to six days following the healing ceremony. Thus, the maximum amount of time for healing, including diet and remedies, is twenty days, providing no serious dis-ease is being attended.

Cost Range

Prices for chants range from $20 to $1,000. Length and complexity of the ceremony defines the fee to be paid. Some consumers have traded or bartered for services, but this is not the norm. Emergency requests are met without advance payment, but exchange is expected in order to complete the chant's cycle. Additionally, cost is modified to the means of the client.

Personal Responsibilities

Perhaps of the greatest concern to Native American people is that all people learn to respect Mother Nature. It is their belief that spiritual disharmony arises when these two components of overall health are discarded. Disease is created in mental, spiritual, and physical realms because energy to and from the earth is blocked. Attention to animal life, air, water, people, and the earth serves to expand man's spiritual cohesiveness, which counteracts dis-ease. Furthermore, energy channels acquire harmonious power from these sources, which are needed for total well-being.

You will have to be "open" to a totally different type of healing method, including such techniques as songs and ceremonies, diagnosis, and treatment leading to cures. Healers are absorbed with dispelling and preventing dis-ease. This is not to say that they do not question the healee. The only comparable explanation is the knowledge that one experiences a different type of life during the days of healing rites, much like entering a convent or monastery. Ceremonies are long and involved and require total concentration.

We are not trying to paint a glorified picture for Indian healers. White Americans are virtually "outsiders" in reservations. Many white visitors tend to think "Poor li'l Indian. What can I do for you?" and are taken by the Indians for exactly what the picture projects—suckers. It's like entering a foreign country where you will more than likely experience culture shock and the desire to "fit in." Just be yourself, state your business, and show the same amount of respect you would want someone to bestow upon you.

Consider the clothing that you wear to a healing ceremony. Some tribal practitioners burn clothes after the cleansing and purification practices and others have them cleaned and returned. You will have to research the healing method so that you will be informed and understand what is to be expected as well as the symbols used in the ceremony. Practitioners will be glad to explain their processes and patient requirements. It will be helpful to ask an attendant to describe the mythical chant before it is sung. All these explanations should occur along with negotiation of fee before the treatment begins. This may relieve any consumer who is worried about the language barrier and will aid in visualization during the rites.

Dietary and life-style changes must be assumed by the consumer. Practitioners of Indian healing set strict practices about diet during and immediately following the healing ceremony. It is felt that after being cleansed, purified, and blessed, one shows respect for the harmonious state of the body by assuming responsibility for what enters it. Because this belief has been symbolically impressed upon the healee during healing rites, it is often left unstated.

Finally, arrangements about date, time, and transportation should be made in advance if at all possible. It will take a lot of time and commitment to make a healing request known to a Native American practitioner, and unfortunately, this is not an easy task. One of the organizations listed in this chapter may point you in the correct direction. The U.S. Indian Health Service tries to employ Native American physicians and they may serve as connecting points. Fees for services should be negotiated before the ceremony and reflect your commitment to healing.

Informational Organizations

Meta Tantay Foundation
PO Box 707
Carlin, NV 89822

Four Directions Foundation
PO Box 188
Carte Madera, CA 94925

Institute for the Development of Indian Law
927 15th Street, NW, Suite 200
Washington, DC 20005

Consistencies

1. Native American practitioners treat spirit, mind, and body through a combination of such natural therapies as fasting, steam treatments, manipulation, massage, and symbolic chants and dances. They are, therefore, holistic practitioners.

2. Healers make use of natural derivatives (herbs) grown and prepared for healing. Side effects are managed by combining the natural observations of the healer with the experience of his or her ancestors.

3. A concentrated effort is aimed at the healee by all of those in attendance at Indian ceremonies. This remarkable social support system affords "extra" psychological reinforcement of healing practices. This is one technique that might play an important part in Western healing.

4. In this method, a waking visualization is enacted so that identification with heroes and heroines is superimposed over the consciousness of the healee. Practitioners, then, present a mythical opportunity in which the healee takes the responsibility of conquering and curing dis-ease. This form of symbolic healing is currently gaining acceptance among contemporary physicians and psychiatrists.

5. Like acupuncture, Native American healers adhere to an ancient philosophy of preventing and maintaining a healthy mind and body. It is this synthesis of physical, mental, and cultural processes that is responsible for the resurgence of the holistic philosophy and the emerging importance of native healers in modern society.

Inconsistencies

1. Counseling on life-style and dietary habits is not available from Indian healers. Consequently, healing is incomplete from the holistic perspective. Although psychotherapy and dietary examples are alluded to in healing ceremonies, no actual interim is devoted to instruction about these aspects.

2. Native Americans believe that all people should be made aware of their personal contributions to peace, health, vitality, and harmonious existence. If this is truly the case, why haven't they tried to imprint these beliefs on society by educating interested people rather than stereotyping all people as having contrary views. A bias seems to emerge in both parties. Furthermore, inquiries about healing from other races are answered only seldomly. Thus, Native Americans are increasing the gap between the two cultures.

3. Only two organizations offer educational programs. White apprentices to the Indian way of knowledge are extremely rare. This severely limits the Native American healing and further adds to deteriorating relations between white and red Americans.

4. Not all Native Americans adhere to the beliefs and practices described in this chapter. Oftentimes, we tend to overgeneralize the customs of Indian healers to apply to all Native Americans. However, just as with any culture, some practice traditional beliefs and others ignore them.

Sources to Read

Atkinson, Donald T. *Magic, Myth, and Medicine.* Cleveland: World Publishing Company, 1956.

Atkinson, M. J. *Indians of the Southwest.* San Antonio, TX: The Naylor Company, 1963.

Bailey, Libert H. *How Plants Got Their Names.* New York: Dover Publications, 1963.

Boyd, Doug. *Rolling Thunder.* New York: Random House, 1974.

Brown, J. W. "Native American Contributions to Science, Engineering, and Medicine," *Science* (1975): Vol. 189, pp. 38–40.

Castaneda, Carlos. *The Eagle's Gift.* New York: Simon and Schuster, 1981.

———. *Tales of Power.* New York: Simon and Schuster, 1974.

Cohen, Felix. "Americanizing the White Man," *The American Scholar* 21, no. 2 (Spring 1952), pp. 177–191.

Coon, Nelson. *An American Herbal: Using Plants for Healing.* New York: Healthside Press, 1963.

Corlett, William Thomas. *The Medicine Man of the American Indian and His Cultural Background.* Springfield, IL: Charles C. Thomas, 1935.

Douglas, William O. "The People of Cades Cove," *National Geographic Magazine* 132, no. 1 (July 1963): 60–95.

Driver, Harold E. *The Americas on the Eve of the Discovery.* Englewood Cliffs,, NJ: Prentice-Hall, 1964.

——. *Indians of North America.* Chicago: University of Chicago Press, 1961.

Dubos, Rene. *Man, Medicine and Environment.* New York: Praeger, 1968.

Dunlop, Richard. *Doctors of the American Frontier.* Garden City, NY: Doubleday, 1965.

Fire, J., and **Erdoes, R.** *Lame Deer: Seeker of Visions.* New York: Simon and Schuster, 1972.

Forbes, Jack D., ed. *The Indian in America's Past.* Englewood Cliffs, NJ: Prentice-Hall, 1964.

Greenlee, Robert F. "Medicine and Curing Practices of the Modern Florida Seminoles," *American Anthropologist* 46, no. 3 (July–September, 1944), pp. 317–328.

Halifox, Joan, Ph.D. *Shamanic Voices, A Survey of Visionary Narratives.* New York: Dutton, 1979.

Hall, Manly P. *Healing: The Divine Art.* Los Angeles: Philosophical Research Society, 1944.

Jarvis, D. C., M.D. *Folk Medicine.* Philadelphia: Lea and Febiger, 1959.

Krippner, Stanley, and **Villoldo, A.** *Realms of Healing.* Millbrae, CA: Celestial Arts, 1976.

Landes, Ruth. "Potawatomi Medicine," *Translations, Kansas Academy of Science* 66, no. 4 (Winter 1963), pp. 553–599.

Maddox, John Lee. *The Medicine Man: A Sociological Study of the Character and Evolution of Shamanism.* New York: Macmillan, 1923.

Mahr, August C. "Materia Medica and Therapy Among the North American Forest Indians," *Ohio State Archaeological and Historical Quarterly* 60, no. 4 (1951), pp. 331–354.

Newcomb, F. J. *Navaho Neighbors.* Norman, OK: University of Oklahoma Press, 1966.

Otto, Herbert A., and **Knight, James W.** (eds.) *Dimensions in Wholistic Healing.* Chicago, IL, 1979.

Radin, Paul. *Autobiography of a Winnebago Indian.* New York: Dover Publications, 1963.

Rands, James Hall. *The North Carolina Indians.* Chapel Hill, NC: University of North Carolina Press, 1963.

Sandner, Donald F. "Navaho Medicine," *Human Nature Magazine,* July, 1978.

Scully, Virginia. *Treasury of American Indian Herbs: Their Lore and Their Use for Food and Medicine.* New York: Crown, 1970.

Slotkin, James S. *The Peyote Religion: A Study in Indian-White Relations.* Glencoe, IL: The Free Press, 1903.

Solomon, Julian H. *The Book of Indian Crafts and Indian Lore.* New York: Harper and Row, 1928.

Thorwald, Jurgen. *Science and Secrets of Early Medicine.* New York: Harcourt Brace and World, 1963.

Underhill, Ruth. *Red Man's America.* Chicago: University of Chicago Press, 1953.

Vogel, Virgil. *Native American Medicine.* Norman, OK: University of Oklahoma Press, 1970.

Waters, Frank. *Book of the Hopi.* New York: Ballantine Books, 1963.

Weiner, Michael A. *Earth Medicine—Earth Foods.* New York: Macmillan, 1972.

Wissler, Clark. *Indians of the United States.* Garden City, NY: Doubleday, 1949.

Wayman, Leland C., and **Bailey, Flora L.** "Two Examples of Navajo Physiotherapy," *American Anthropologist* 46, no. 3 (July–September 1944), pp. 329–337.

11

HERBALISM

Definition

One of the major medicines of days past that is currently being revived is the art and science of herbalism. The popularity of scientific evidence supporting Chinese cures through the use of herbs (the "barefoot doctors") has helped spur this "underground" practice and has led some to endorse this as an emerging method in the field of public health (Lee, 1978). All of this is due to a renewed interest by consumers in natural alternatives for treatment of dis-ease. You may already be aware of the fact that Native Americans and early settlers relied upon roots, herbs, leaves, and barks as major sources of vitamins and minerals, and also used these substances for cures. In the more recent past our grandparents grew many "simple" herbs in their gardens in order to have an accessible, fresh supply for use in preventing and treating dis-ease.

Holistic herbalists, as much as any holistic health method contained in this book, are involved in a swirl of controversy between modern and ancient science. Nicholas Culpeper (1616–1654), an English physician, was involved in a similar debate between scientific traditions. Culpeper was profiled in the *Journal of the American Medical Association* in 1964. In 1649 Culpeper published the *Pharmacopoeia* of the Royal College of Physicians. His colleagues were angry because Culpeper disclosed their "secret" formulas by translating them from Latin. In a critique of his associates, he said he had a vision that was dictated to him by his conscience, nothing supernatural, but which showed the following:

> All the sick People in *England* presented themselves before me, and told me, They had Herbs in their Gardens that might cure them, but knew not the Vertues of them: They praid me (for God's sake, and as I would answer it another day) that I would help them; For the *Colledg of Physitians* were so *Proud, so Surly,* and so *Covetous,* that Honesty went a begging in *Amen-Corner,* and could find no entertainment. [Cited in *JAMA* 187 (11, 1964): 167; from the third edition of *A Physical Directory: Or A Translation of the Dispensatory Made by the Colledg of Physitians of London, And by them imposed upon all the Apothecaries of England to Make up their Medicines By* (London: P. Cole, 1651)]

Culpeper, along with other doctors of his time, were not only physicians but were also herbalists and astrologers. During his life he translated other classic medical works such as Galen's *Art of Physic* for use in English medicine. In his day Culpeper translated what he considered to be a systematic or "scientific" classification system for using herbs to prevent disease. It had been passed down from the Arabs, the Greeks, and the Romans. Using this system, he could ascertain what planets caused the dis-ease, what part of the body was afflicted with the dis-ease, and what herbs were associated with both planetary influence and dis-ease.

The theory involved both opposites and similars or sympathies. The dis-eases could be opposed by the herbs of the planet opposite to the planet that caused them. For instance, the herbs of Mercury were associated with the brain and the herbs of Jupiter with the breast and the liver. When using herbs to oppose the dis-eases of Jupiter (breast), he would recommend herbs of Mercury, which also represented the brain. When using the sympathetic method, he would administer herbs with properties similar to the dis-ease or, for example, those of Jupiter with a liver dis-ease.

In the *English Physician Enlarged,* published in 1653, Culpeper provided a list of the botanicals, their place of growth, the time of the year when they matured, their preparation for use and the dis-eases for which they were valuable. It was two centuries before English replaced Latin as the official medical language in English medicine, which means that his books influenced medicine until the 1820s (See "Nicholas

Culpeper" in *The Dictionary of Natural Biography*, vol. 5 [Oxford: Oxford University Press, 1959–1960]).

Thus, herbs are an integral part of the heritage of medicine. In fact, according to Paul Lee, Ph.D., the executive director of the Herb Trade Association, in an interview in *Well-Being* (issue 34), it was not until 1828, when a German chemist named Wohler artificially synthesized urea, when the "distinction between inorganic, natural, and synthetic broke down." With the reintroduction of holistic health in medicine, one finds the reemergence of the controversy between the modern physicalists, who believe in mechanisms of the physical body, and the vitalists who credit the Life Force. Herbalism, therefore, is not a science according to the modern definition of that term. It is a precursor of modern drug treatment. Many of the medications developed by synthetic means in the modern drug industry grew out of experiments with natural herbs.

Herbs, then, are grounded in nature. This basic belief of herbalists forms the foundation for their practice. Like Native American healers, herbalists explain that the energy forces within nature are present in nature's "fruits" and can be strengths from which individuals draw energy to realign, balance, or heal the body. Herbs discharge their energy within the body and deliver their potent effects on more than one level at a time. Holistic herbalists maintain that for every sickness there exists a cure within nature. Likewise, herbal professionals suggest that botanicals, in order to be life-giving, must be extracted from their natural environment. The fresher the herb, the more potent is its qualities. Practitioners do not often make use of "man-made" substances within individual remedies.

We caution the reader not to stereotype herbalists as being confined only to ethnic groups or such economically deprived rural areas as Appalachia. Stekert (1970) found that people from Appalachia who had moved to Detroit still maintained their practices. When we were interviewing herbalists, we found that many practiced in urban areas, especially where traditional customs were still in vogue. In San Francisco's Chinatown, for example, herbal shops flourish. In the last ten years modern, urbanized Americans have brought about an explosion in the use of herbs for diet and medicinal purposes.

Obviously, herbalism, like any other practice, whether considered scientific or nonscientific, is based upon beliefs in which people have faith. Modern science and medicine are based upon faith in statistical reasoning and technological procedures. Modern herbalists require faith in the self-regulating properties of the body, the vital force, and the ability of herbs to affect these processes. However, in order to maintain a critical stance, we believe it is best to define herbalism as an art rather than a science.

Holistic herbalists are, in a sense, much like gourmet cooks, mixing and matching concoctions of varying amounts, tastes, and energies so that the prescription will be suited for the whole individual. As such, mixing preparations, practitioners assert, must be individualized in order to meet specific needs of the client so as to "ignite" the self-regulating processes of the body.

"Essences" are substances that have been reduced from the whole plant to an oil. We found that some herbalists feel that these are more potent than teas or tonics for affecting the vital force. Like homoeopaths, these practitioners believe that the pure extract spurs faster and more complete action within the body. Herbal botanicals are usually categorized according to reactions in the body. Many of these remedies will sound familiar to readers, since they are often medicinals found in drugs stores today. Some of the major classifications and examples of each are provided in the following box:

Herbal Classifications

CLASSIFICATION	REACTION	EXAMPLES
Alternatives	Gradually alter a condition	black cohosh root yellow dock root
Astringents	Tighten skin or mucous membranes	white oak bark shepherd's purse herb
Bitter tonics	Stimulate saliva and gastric juice	calumba wild cherry bark
Bland dietetics	Nonirritating, nutritive	slippery elm okra pods
Calmatives	Mild calming effect	fennel seed sage herb
Cathartics	Cleanse bowels	goldenseal ginger
Diuretics	To increase urine flow	parsley root wild carrot herb
Emetics	To produce vomiting	bayberry bark boneset
Expectorants	To expel phlegm	white pine yerba santa herb
Nervines	To relax	camomile yarrow
Refrigerants	Cooling beverages	red clover herb peppermint
Sedatives	Sleep-inducing, pain relief	vervdin herb hops
Stimulants	To increase responses	cayenne sweet gum herb

The various mixtures of botanicals depend upon the herbalist's interpretation of the actions of herbs and the individual's complaint. Premixed remedies usually contain three parts of the healing herb to one part herb for taste, one part herb for protective properties, and one part laxative. Other remedies consist of simply making a tea by steeping the healing herb in clean, fresh water.

Some of the holistic herbalists we interviewed told us that herbs can be used for reasons other than their curative properties. They assert that vitamins and minerals are manufactured within plants. Vitamin A, for example, can be found in alfalfa, and Vitamin C is obtained from rose hips. Calcium is provided by camomile and chives. They emphasize that vitamins and minerals that exist in plants are easier to digest than when they are derived from fish or animals. These practitioners also maintain that there are botanical sources for hormones such as pleurisy root, sarsaparilla, and wheat germ. These beliefs assume that nature is the source of preventive health in addition to the treatment of symptoms.

A point of contention among herbal practitioners is the use of parts of plants versus the whole plant. Professionals within the field are divided. Many point out that specific parts of plants are more valuable for relief, therefore only that part should be put to use in a remedy. For example, the leaves of mullein are often put to use for coughs. On the other hand, other practitioners support the belief that the whole plant is needed for an effective cure. It is their contention that the vital elements within the whole plant ensure proper integration of the herb within the body. As Leslie Kaslof (1978)* explains, "Whole plant substances . . . make available, in concentrated form, a vital force—activity sufficient to catalyze a revitalizing biochemical response." Furthermore, those practitioners who employ the whole plant report that those who use only parts must "make up the difference" with additional herbal remedies.

You may be wondering how herbalists are licensed to practice. Though they attend medical schools like other physicians in such countries as England and China, herbalism is against the law in the United States. Herbal practitioners are forbidden from diagnosing or treating dis-ease. In fact, they cannot even use the words! This is in spite of the fact that licensed naturopaths, homoeopaths, and allopaths can employ herbs for treatment of dis-ease. Since they are not regulated, we recommend that consumers interested in herbalism sign an informed consent form when visiting a practitioner. However, legally, neither

*Excerpt from *Wholistic Dimensions in Healing: A Resource Guide* by Leslie J. Kaslof. Copyright © 1978 Leslie J. Kaslof. Reprinted by permission of Doubleday and Company.

healer nor healee is protected under the law. The healer can still be arrested for practicing medicine without a license, and the healee has no legal recourse in the case of malpractice.

Nutrition plays a small role in all holistic practices. A well-balanced diet ensures a faster cure, according to herbalists. Nutrition instruction given by herbalists is focused upon consumption of foods close to their natural state. An important point here is that practitioners intend that clients become aware of foods that counteract herbal properties. In fact, some herbalists feel that foods high in protein produce body reactions that are counterproductive to most botanicals. We also found that many herbalists support the consumption of lean meats.

Relaxation, massage, manipulation, and exercise are other supportive measures offered by some herbalists. However, not all practitioners make use of these methods within their herbal practice. Actually, few of the herbalists we interviewed had expertise in these areas, even though knowledge about the subjects was suggested or implied by their comments. For example, an herbalist may suggest that a client work outside frequently and walk a lot or pray and meditate daily. However, these suggestions were secondary to the concern for herbs and adequate nutrition and were not part of an organized therapy program.

Two important findings related to practicing herbalists were that healees had not previously been cured by conventional medical treatment and they *believed* that the herbal healer would cure them. Clients also alleged that visiting an herbalist made them feel more at ease in discussing problems associated with the dis-ease as opposed to when they visited normal physicians. This "personal appeal" created by the practitioner appeared to reinforce the client's belief in the cure.

When compared with other holistic healers in this book, there are very few practicing herbalists. Even though England and Canada have well-established groups of medical herbalists and herbal institutions, the U.S. does not. Though there are physicians who employ herbal remedies in combination with other treatment measures, a large proportion of these have been absorbed into somewhat more "accepted" fields, such as naturopathy and homoeopathy. Unless he or she is widely acknowledged in the field of herbal medicine, those who are not part of a medical structure do not advertise their profession. This makes it difficult for interested consumers to locate an herbal practitioner. We found that area herbal societies are most often aware of those knowledgeable in herbal remedies. "Word of mouth" appears to be the most efficient method for finding a holistic herbalist.

We believe that herbalism represents an incomplete holistic model due to the lack of an individualized health maintenance program and other holistic elements. However, there are some definite assets to a holistic herbal practice. Practitioners point out that activation of the body, mind, and spirit is a natural or inherent ability within each of us. If one is unable to raise the self-healing properties, practitioners assert that only natural means work to enhance them. They also affirm that natural measures are forms of "assistance" to the body, since healing is the patient's responsibility.

Type of Healing

Because of the measures employed by herbal practitioners, we feel that herbalism is a natural healing modality. There is, however, some question about certain botanicals frequently used by herbalists. As we reported earlier, many current drugs are based on properties found in herbs. For this reason alone consumers should thoroughly investigate a recommended substance before it is consumed. Do not let this scare you away from this healing method; just be cautious. Relatively few herbal substances are dangerous.

Recently (June 1979), the American Holistic Medical Association reported "side effects" of some herbal substances. Effects of these range from diarrhea and sodium retention to hallucination and heart failure. They recommend that large doses of teas of the following herbs be employed cautiously:

horsetail grass	buckthorn bark	senna
burdock	catnip	juniper
hydrangea	lobelia	cassava
jimsonweed	wormwood	nutmeg
camomile	goldenrod	marigold
yarrow	Saint-John's-wort	licorice root
Devil's claw root	pennyroyal oil	sassafras root
ginseng	mandrake root	snakeroot
mistletoe	poke	matè tea
	indian tobacco	

and seeds, pits, barks, or leaves of the following:

apricot	bitter almond	cherry
chokecherry	peach	pear
apple	plum	cassava beans

Holistic herbalists do employ many of the herbs in the AHMA's list. For example, yarrow, they point out, is an excellent tea for colds and fevers unless the client has a history of allergies. However, pennyroyal oil has been found to induce spontaneous abortions and has led to fatalities.

Herbalists maintain that a complete makeup of the healee's history is needed in order to prevent such detrimental side effects as these. Additionally, individual reactions to herbal medicaments are studied carefully by responsible practitioners in order to avoid problems of this nature. Once again, you can see that the controversy surrounding herbalists is a crucial factor in seeking their advice. In order to avoid these problems, please see our recommendations in the conclusion of the book.

Holistic herbalists express that individuals who make use of herbs on a regular basis support many varied uses for them other than their nutritional and medicinal functions. A large number of practitioners teach "simpling" to encourage the diversified use of these substances. In addition to being used in cooking, herbs can also be employed for food coloring, cosmetics, dyeing, and for quitting smoking. For the client, this practice symbolizes nature's interdependence with man and vice versa. According to professionals, if an herb needs water, food, air, and sunlight for growth and healthy appearance, then so does the human. Nurturing plants can also be a satisfying hobby or avocation.

Following is a list we have composed of herbs and their reported uses. We stress that any reader wishing to make use of these or any other botanical read up on its history. Often herbs have more than one medicinal use, one of which may not be a complementary effect. Although we were unable to find information that pinpointed specific side effects of these substances, that does not mean they will not cause serious reactions. As a general rule, practitioners recommend one teaspoon of powdered herb or one tablespoon of dried herb to two cups of boiling water. Steep this mixture for twenty minutes before drinking as a tea. One-half cup of the tincture, according to herbalists, should be consumed four times a day so that a new solution is made fresh daily. Discontinue use of herbal preparations after one week.

HERB	REPORTED USE
Rosemary, willow	headache
Cayenne, gentian	indigestion
Angelica, lemons	prevention and well-being
Skullcap, hops	pain
Wintergreen, red sage	fever
Ground ivy, horehound	stimulation of perspiration
Mullein, coltsfoot	coughs and colds
Ginger, Blue Flag	constipation
Valerian, Red Clover	relaxation

Renewed interest among some scientific organizations is leading to thorough testing of botanical substances that according to folklore can treat such dis-eases as heart disease and hypertension. Until the "scientific evidence" is published, little is known about how herbs work or why. A forerunner of the research on herbs is the Herb Trade Association, a professional association for buyers, pharmacists, biochemists, and many others. Through cooperative research efforts, their findings will likely expand our current understanding of herbal actions and reactions. Although some physicians make use of herbal remedies, they do not have data that meet the specifications of the entire scientific community. Presently, however, responsible herbalists point out that we will have to rely upon extensive case histories to demonstrate that herbal remedies do activate the individual's self-healing abilities.

Description of Healing Method

The first visit to a holistic herbalist may take a lot of time, as long as two hours, since there are many aspects to be taken into consideration before herbs are recommended. Legitimate herbalists request information about diet, physical activity, daily routine, feelings and desires, surroundings, job activities, and personal friends. Because holistic herbalists think in terms of the whole person, questions should be personal and detailed. Each remedy is highly individualized in order to affect the total state of the individual as interpreted by the herbalist. Nutritional and environmental changes are most often designed by both the practitioner and healee, although some herbalists only recommend changes. Counseling and alterations of the outlined changes drawn up by the practitioner and client take place in subsequent visitations. Additionally, botanical advice is reevaluated and often altered.

Practitioners recommend herbs as powdered or dried mixtures, oils, ointments, lotions, extracts, or tinctures. Powdered and dried mixtures can be taken as a tea or put into gelatin capsules. Extracts and tinctures are liquid in form and can be mixed with juice or taken separately. Ointments, lotions, and oils are frequently ready for immediate use. By and large, practitioners supply healees with the substances or mixtures required, but occasionally one is referred to a distributor or a specific store.

Whole plants reduced to their "essence" are used to make extracts or oils. Powdered or dried herbs may either be parts of plants or whole plant substances, depending upon the herbalist's preference. Ask the herbalist for his or her own preference and see if it agrees with yours. This is because herbalists assert that while taking parts of plants, it is crucial that one eat correctly. Proper diet, then, assures that secondary actions that may be lost by only taking part of the plant are compensated for by adequate nutrition. Most herbalists believe that the whole plant is most beneficial because the secondary effects of catalyzing and/or balancing are present. In either case, proper diet will provide one with extra benefits in the assimilation of herbal medicaments in the body.

The curative effects of herbal remedies take longer to notice than the effects of such over-the-counter drugs as laxatives, nasal sprays, and cold tablets. Previous clients tell us that the effects of tinctures and extracts may be noticed after three days. The effects of herbal teas and capsules seem slower but are usually recognized in three to five days. Relief from botanical lotions and ointments, however, is felt immediately. They "work about the same as any you can buy in a drugstore," as one person told us. Herbal practitioners feel that even though herbs are slower acting than drugs, they do work if the client holds on to the faith he or she places in the remedy, the healer, and the recuperative abilities of the body.

We discovered that a few holistic herbalists examine the belief systems and attitudes of the healee. According to practitioners, faith is the most important factor in healing. Beliefs that "it won't work" inhibit the curative powers of herbs, the healer, and the individual. Although symptoms of dis-ease may fade, holistic herbalists try to instill in clients the idea that the cause of the symptoms must also be dissolved. Practitioners point out that counseling a client after herbal treatment can influence changes toward health and well-being by resolving conflicts. It is this fact that gives herbalism its almost "occult" qualities. It is the hope of these professionals that as a body begins to heal itself, less "help" would be required from the healer or a botanical remedy because the client would be aware of his or her own healing processes. In the long run, it is the client, they assert, who decides to put self-healing qualities to work in a positive and health-giving manner.

Diseases Treated

There have been many books written on dis-eases that have reportedly been cured or prevented by herbs. It is impossible to list all of them here, but we have included some of the most common ones. See the sources listed at the end of this chapter for those not listed here. Some of these diseases are aches, abscesses, fever, bladder and bowel troubles, blood poisoning, burns, bleeding, boils, cancer, coughs, colds, colic, diabetes, dandruff, earache, eye problems, fainting, gas, goiter, gout, prostate trouble, hay fever, headaches, blood pressure, itches, kidney problems, pleurisy, phlegm, pain, relaxation problems, sinus, stings, swellings, sprains and strains, sores, toothaches, tumors, tobacco habit, ulcers, warts, and wounds.

Duration of Treatment

Unfortunately, in spite of all the practitioners' talk of "holism," very few herbalists spend the amount of time with a healee required to integrate holistic methods into the treatment period. But those few who do include holistic measures point out that since herbal remedies are natural and are usually suggested in much smaller amounts, the potent effects are delivered subtly and therefore take longer than other healing methods. However, if the healee is in pain, herbs are often advised in larger quantities and effects may be felt sooner.

According to health practitioners, if one has had an ear infection for six months, he or she can expect relief from an herbal remedy in a lesser period of time. A cure, however, is much slower, usually taking approximately six weeks. Herbal practitioners espouse that the longer one has been ill, the longer it will take one to get well. The following is a general rule to follow for duration of herbal treatment and cure: It takes one week to cure for every month of dis-ease. The duration of treatment, according to previous clients, is commonly one week to six weeks. Most previous clients report that they remained under the herbalist's care for at least four weeks. This allowed practitioners to adjust herbal medicaments, suggest personal changes, and counsel the healee. If one is impatient for a cure, herbalism is not for you.

Cost Range

Herbalism is one of the least expensive of the healing methods we have reviewed. The cost of prepackaged teas may vary if one purchases them in health food stores, but most herbalists supply necessary botanicals for treatment. Fees are based upon whether or not the herb was purchased, picked, grown, or a prepared concoction, in addition to the client's ability to pay. Some of these costs are listed here.

Initial visit—donation to $20
Follow-up visit—donation to $10
Stock solutions—$1–$7
Teas—$1–$8
Oils, extracts, scents, tinctures—$1.75–$15 (1 oz. to 1 gal.)
Liniments—$1.75–$3 (4 oz. to 8 oz.)
Single bulk packs of herbs—$.50–$9 (1 oz. to 16 oz.)
Single herb capsules—$3.15–$14.50 (per 100)
Herbal combination capsules—$3.45–$23.70 (per 100) (usually two)
Plants—$.10–$7.50
Seeds—$.05–$.50
Salves—$.50–$1.50

Personal Responsibilities

As a client, you should keep several points in mind when seeing a holistic herbal practitioner. He or she will ask many personal questions and you are encouraged to answer all of these honestly. In order to assure that medicaments meet the specifications of the entire system and side effects are averted, the full cooperation of the client is required to obtain detailed personal information.

It is the responsibility of the client to adhere to botanical recommendations in order to obtain relief from the symptoms of dis-ease. This is also true of nutritional suggestions made by the herbalist. Compliance with a practitioner's suggestions is important in any healing field, but it is especially vital in herbalism. Medicinals are highly diluted and must be consumed with regularity in order to affect your self-healing processes. Likewise, proper dietary intake is crucial to the integration of herbs into the body as well as in the individual as a whole.

The maintenance of health and well-being is exclusively the consumer's responsibility. In most herbal practices, we found no structured design presented for clients to follow when treatment is complete. As a result, consumers must draw up their own plan by "reading between the lines," so to speak, and implement this plan into their living style.

Remember that there are no certification, formal training, or licensing procedures in this country. Exercise caution when you visit an herbalist. Though "world of mouth" is the most effective way to contact an herbalist, make certain that your sources are reliable. Along these lines, inquire into the background of the healer and find out how effective his or her methods have been with other patients. These guidelines are extremely important, since herbalism is illegal.

Informational Organizations

Herb Trade Association
PO Box 409
Santa Cruz, CA 95016

International Institute for Biological and Botanical Research, Ltd.
PO Box 912
Brooklyn, NY 11202

Society for Economic Botany, Inc.
Department of Pharmacognosy and Pharmacology
833 South Wood Street
Chicago, IL 60612

Medicine Wheel
PO Box 1211
Idyllwild, CA 92349

Consistencies

1. The holistic herbalist should examine environmental, psychological, spiritual, mental, and physical aspects of dis-ease before suggesting a botanical remedy to affect inherent healing abilities. When practiced in this manner, herbalism is consistent with the principles of holistic health.

2. Nutrition is a focus of responsible herbal care. Dietary recommendations include increased water intake and foods consumed closer to their natural state as the primary components of nutritional education.

3. Herbalists are much less expensive than most other holistic practitioners. Herbal medicaments are inexpensive and available from the practitioner.

4. The holistic philosophy of inherent healing abilities and energy forces within nature is put to use in herbal medicine. Energy from herbs is viewed as a cooperator with innate self-healing processes—one supports the other. Herbalists propose that natural abilities to heal are aided by natural forces within herbs.

5. Health strategies during treatment should be designed by the healee and practitioner operating as a team. It is hoped that clients will adapt this plan to their life-style after treatment.

6. The "herbal renaissance" is an important aspect of the humanizing trend in modern medicine. Herbalists describe their profession as a synthesis of man and nature rather than the blind dogma of controlling and conquering nature. This call for a return to more traditional forms of treatment is further evidence that the holistic model is based on a classical view of health and dis-ease wherein the individual views life as a cooperative venture between many levels of existence.

Inconsistencies

1. Herbalism, as mentioned already, is involved in a scientific controversy between the physicalists and vitalists. Around 1820 the vitalists lost their power to the physicalists, when it was learned that drugs could be synthesized. In the early 1970s, this controversy reemerged when the unnecessary side effects of drug therapy became evident. While herbalism's belief in the natural healing processes of the body is consistent with holism, the recency of its reemergence has left it open to criticism, since it has not yet been able to formalize itself to incorporate the examination, treatment, and creation of health in a form easily implemented into the everyday life of the individual.

2. Herbal experts are divided into several occupational types, such as distributors of products, healers, aromatics experts, growers, exporters, biochemists, and pharmacologists. One must be careful to choose the type of professional needed since there are no professional organizations certified as the "official" institutions of this field.

3. Herbal remedies are only preventive or suggestive. By law herbalists are not allowed to say that herbal methods are diagnostic or remedies are cures.

4. There is no health reconstruction plan for the client to follow when treatment is complete. This part of the "cure" is left entirely up to the consumer. While there is a yearly conference of herbalists conducted by the Herb Trade Association, it is difficult for the majority of interested consumers to afford the travel expenses necessary to attend.

5. There is much confusion among herbalists about whether parts of plants or whole plants should be employed as medicaments. This indicates that there is confusion in the "art" of herbalism. Such division among experts only further separates herbalism from other holistic fields. In order for herbal medicine to become more than a "secondary" area in healing, this would first have to be resolved within the field.

6. It appears that fresh botanicals, rather than dried or powdered, would best meet "natural law" specifications. It is general practice, however, to make use of dried and/or powdered herbs. This seems to contradict the herbalists' belief that "the fresher the herb, the more potent" are its properties.

7. Some herbs are considered dangerous. Consumers should research any botanical and become aware of its benefits and deficits before it is ingested, and they should exercise caution by not overindulging in herbal treatments.

Sources to Read

Bach, Edward. *Heal Thyself.* London: Daniel, 1946.

——. *The Twelve Healers and Other Remedies.* London: Fowler, 1964.

Bianchini, Francesco, and **Corbetta, F.** *Health Plants of the World: Atlas of Medicinal Plants.* New York: Newsweek, 1977.

British Herbal Pharmacopoeia. London: British Herbal Medicine Association, 1971.

Buchman, Diane D. *Complete Herbal Guide to Natural Health and Beauty.* Garden City, NY: Doubleday, 1973.

Carter, Mary Ellen, and **McGarey, W.** *Edgar Cayce on Healing.* New York: Warner, 1972.

Cerney, J. V. *Handbook of Unusual and Unorthodox Healing Methods.* Englewood Cliffs, NJ: Prentice-Hall, 1976.

Chancellor, Phillip M., ed. *Handbook of the Bach Flower Remedies.* London: Daniel, 1971.

Christopher, John. *School of Natural Healing.* Provo, UT: BiWorld, 1976.

Clark, Linda A. *Get Well Naturally.* New York: Arco, 1968.

——. *Handbook of Natural Remedies for Common Ailments.* Old Greenwich, CT: Devin-Adair, 1976.

Culpeper, Nicholas. *Culpeper's English Physician and Complete Herbal Remedies.* North Hollywood, CA: Wilshire Book Co., 1972.

Elbert, Virginia, and **Elbert, G.** *Fun with Growing Herbs Indoors.* New York: Crown, 1974.

Fluck, Hans. *Medicinal Plants.* Slough, England: Foulsham, 1976.

Foster, Gertrude B. *Herbs for Every Garden.* New York: Dutton, 1973.

Gabriel, Engrid. *Herb Identifier and Handbook.* New York: Sterling, 1975.

Geographical Health Studies Program for the John E. Fogarty International Center for Advanced Study in the Health Sciences. *A Barefoot Doctor's Manual.* Washington, D.C.: U.S. Department of Health, Education and Welfare, 1974.

Grieve, Maude. *A Modern Herbal. Vol. I and II.* New York: Dover, 1971.

Hammond, Sally. *We Are All Healers.* New York: Ballantine, 1974.

Harris, Ben Charles. *The Complete Herbal.* Barre, MA: Barre Publishing Co., 1972.

——. *Eat the Weeds.* New York: Barre Publishing Co., 1972.

Harris, Lloyd. *The Book of Garlic.* New York: Holt, Rinehart and Winston, 1975.

Hewlett-Parsons, James. *Herbs, Health, and Healing.* Northants, England: Thorsons, 1975.

Hun-nan Chung i yao yen chin so. *A Barefoot Doctor's Manual.* Philadelphia: Running Press, 1977.

Hyde, Frederick Fletcher. *The Origin and Practice of Herbal Medicine.* Leicester, England: National Institute of Medical Herbalists, 1978.

Jarvis, EdForest C., M.D. *Folk Medicine.* Greenwich, CT: Fawcett World, 1976.

Kadans, Joseph M. *Encyclopedia of Fruits, Vegetables, Nuts and Seeds for Healthful Living.* Los Angeles: Prentice-Hall, 1973.

——. *Encyclopedia of Medicinal Herbs.* New York: Arco, 1970.

——. *Modern Encyclopedia of Herbs.* Englewood Cliffs, NJ: Prentice-Hall, 1970.

Kaslof, Leslie J. *Herb and Ailment Cross Reference Chart.* Brooklyn, NY: United Communications, 1972.

——. *Wholistic Dimensions in Healing.* Garden City, NY: Doubleday, 1978.

Kloss, Jethro. *Back to Eden.* Santa Barbara, CA: Woodbridge Press, 1975.

Kreig, Margaret B. *Green Medicine: The Search for Plants That Heal.* Chicago: Rand McNally and Co., 1964.

Krockmal, Arnold and **Connie.** *Guide to Medicinal Plants of the U.S.* New York: Quadrangle, 1973.

LaDean, Griffin. *Herbs to the Rescue.* Provo, UT: BiWorld Publishers, 1976.

Law, Donald. *Herb Growing for Health.* New York: Arco, 1972.

Lee, Dr. Paul. "The Herb Renaissance: Can Science Return to Nature?" *Well Being Magazine,* 34, 1978, pp. 32 to 38.

Lewis, Walter, and **Lewis, E.** *Medical Botany: Plants Affecting Man's Health.* New York: Wiley Interscience, 1973.

Li, Chen Pien. *Chinese Herbal Medicine.* Washington, DC: U.S. Government Printing Office, 1974.

Lucas, Richard. *Common and Uncommon Uses of Herbs for Healthful Living.* New York: Arco, 1970.

——. *Secrets of the Chinese Herbalists.* Englewood Cliffs, NJ: Prentice-Hall, 1977.

Lust, John. *The Herb Book.* New York: Benedict Lust, 1974.

Medsger, Oliver. *Edible Wild Plants.* New York: Macmillan, 1963.

Messegue, Maurice. *Way to Natural Health and Beauty.* New York: Macmillan, 1974.

Meyer, Clarence. *American Folk Medicine.* New York: Crowell, 1973.

Meyer, Joseph E. *The Herbalist.* Glenwood, IL: Meyer Books, 1976.

Millspaugh, Charles F. *American Medicinal Plants.* New York: Dover, 1974.

Morton, Julia F., *Folk Remedies of the Low Country.* Miami, FL: E. A. Seemann, 1974.

Rau, Henrietta. *Healing with Herbs.* New York: Arco, 1968.

Reilly, Harold H., and **Brod, R. H.** *Edgar Cayce Handbook for Health Through Drugless Therapy.* Macmillan, 1975.

Rose, Jeanne. *Herbs and Things.* New York: Grosset and Dunlap, 1974.

——. *Jeanne Rose's Herbal Body Book.* New York: Grosset and Dunlap, 1976.

Shook, Edward E. *Elementary Treatise in Herbology.* Lakemont, CA: CSA Press, 1974.

Stekert, E. J. "Focus for Conflict: Southern Mountain Medical Beliefs in Detroit," *Journal of American Folklore,* 83, 1970, pp. 115 to 126.

Weeks, Nora, and **Bullen, V.** *Bach Flower Remedies.* London: Daniel, 1964.

Wheeler, F. J. *The Bach Remedies Repertory.* London: Daniel, 1953.

Weiner, Michael A., Ph.D. *Earth Medicine—Earth Foods: Plant Remedies, Drugs and Natural Foods of the North American Indians.* New York: Macmillan, 1972.

——. *Weiner's Herbal: The Guide to Herb Medicine.* New York: Stein and Day, 1979.

Wren, Richard C., ed. *Potter's New Cyclopedia of Medicinal Herbs and Preparations.* New York: Harper and Row, 1972.

12

BODY THERAPY

Definition

Though we may not be aware of it, most of us have experienced body therapy at one time or another. Rubbing stiff and aching muscles, smoothing the temples for headaches, and applying pressure to bruises to prevent them from blueing are all ways that body therapy is used unknowingly. Although we are not consciously aware that these are body therapies, we know from self-experimentation that these methods have helped soothe and ease pain as well as provide loving and helpful support.

Massage was first practiced by the "founding fathers" of medicine. It is said that Hippocrates required each of his students to learn the mechanics of massage. Massage dwindled until Peter Ling compiled all of the varied methods into the *Swedish massage* (Reilly and Brod, 1975). Since that time many others (Gram, Zander, Reich, and Rolf among others) have contributed to the expansion of massage into body therapy.

Vibrating machines, manipulation, finger pressure, rotations, and many other techniques have also been added to massage. With each new addition to massage therapy, another branch of the healing science is created. For example, chiropractic and osteopathy found massage methods extremely useful within their own modes of healing.

A holistic massage systematically strokes, manipulates, and exercises the body in many ways. Stroking, palming, kneading, friction, pressure, slapping, chopping, and many other "hands on" methods are employed to promote stimulation or relaxation of the skin, nerves, and muscles. Practitioners within the body therapies believe that they adjust energy levels so that the client maintains a balanced physical system. Therapy can be applied to the whole body, as in shiatsu massage, to parts of the body, as in reflexology, or to segments or units of the body, as in rolfing. The various extensions of massage differ in their specific procedures. On the other hand, their underlying reasoning is closely related. Regardless of the body method employed by the therapist, their aim is to affect the self-healing abilities of the receiver.

Though a few areas of body therapy also include dietary emphasis, exercise, and client education, the majority of them do not. In fact, practitioners are quick to point out that body therapy or massage is not a cure: It is only part of a prevention system, an adjunct to other therapy or an energy adjustment method. It is never a singular healing modality. Holistic body therapists consider themselves teachers who open clients to their own self-healing abilities.

Currently within medicine, massage therapy is primarily used for treatment by trained physical therapists. However, unless there is a specific problem, such as a broken limb, physical therapy is confined to an institution such as a hospital, nursing home, ambulatory care unit or a healing spa. So-called health clubs and gyms employ massage therapists—or at least someone trained to give a "rubdown." Often the masseurs and masseuses in health clubs and gyms have not been trained in holistic techniques of massage. Holistic massage techniques involve therapist-receiver concentration, personal attention, and energy exchange in addition to the "hands-on" method.

According to holistic therapists, massage affects energy channels. Any combination of methods is employed to move vital energy through the channels to balance, tone, exercise, stimulate, relax, and strengthen the body. Muscles, connective tissues, glands, organs, skin, blood flow, and hormonal secretions are affected by massage and body therapy techniques. All therapeutic methods attempt to release dis-ease–causing tension and physical strain from (within) the body. However, the expressed purpose of a therapy is not to heal, but rather to help the body heal itself. Although we found some methods that claim to diagnose and treat dis-ease, therapists cannot legally diagnose or treat specific dis-eases unless he or she is an M.D.

The hands of a body therapist are as important as a pilot's eyes. Practitioners explain that much practice is involved in correct hand or finger movements and smooth transitions between strokes. Therapists learn to locate imbalance and defects by touch and correct these with specific method(s). Therapist and receiver are connected through touch, allowing an energy exchange. A master therapist knows up to seventy strokes and makes use of ten or more types of movements with virtually no inconvenience being noticeable to the receiver. Holistic therapists proclaim that a practitioner who is not "tuned into" his or her hands will have little effect on the receiver. Furthermore, those who do not project a caring attitude can cause more damage than good by actually creating energy blocks.

Therapies that are of expert quality fully exercise all muscles by varied hand or finger motions. Harold Reilly, M.D., says that a forty-five minute massage equals four hours of sleep (Reilly and Brod, 1975). The therapist has detailed knowledge of anatomy and is therefore able to "spot" tensions and/or distortions. Although each system has different procedures or movements for the purpose of manipulating energies, all make use of similar philosophical theories. It would be another book altogether to list and describe each method or all the types of therapies related to massage. (Interested consumers will find that sources are available and are listed at the end of this chapter.) To acquaint you with the most popular massage and body therapies in holism, we present their particular therapy strategies following the definition.

A common experience shared by those who have made use of massage or body therapy is an intense emotional release. This is more common in some methods than in others. However, holistic practitioners attribute this to tension released when techniques are applied to the receiver's body. Because years of stress may have built up in a specific area, liberation of that pressure through body therapy frees the energy associated with it. Therapists assert that emotional reactions are expected, and holistic therapists explain that such reactions should be encouraged when they occur. For example, if one cries or "shakes" during a massage, the therapist will stop the treatment (yet remain in contact) until one is finished. In Reichian therapy, this emotional release can also be a carthartic process recalling memories that provided the original source of strain. Therefore, emotional responses are "good" to holistic body therapists and often rid the body of long-standing mental conflicts.

It is also common that flatulence will occur during massage and that one will feel physically tired after therapy has been completed.

Massage practitioners point out that vital energy is rearranged so that it flows freely through areas that have not been receiving the proper amount. However, rearranging the receiver's energy only causes listlessness for a short period of time. Most therapists feel that their particular type of method is a maintenance or preventive system. Practitioners also teach their clients to perform the method at home.

Passive exercise is an integrative part of any holistic massage treatment and should not be eliminated from a practitioner's procedure. Rotation and manipulation are the primary motions therapists employ to accomplish passive exercise. Polarity teachers, reflexologists, and massage therapists contend that movement through passive exercise often alerts the practitioner to energy blocks within the receiver. For example, many joggers are tender around the knee area. According to holistic therapists, after the knee has been massaged, bending the leg so that the calf and thigh meet and rotating the leg at the knee often produce more flexibility and strength. During a complete massage, passive exercise will be put to work where each part of the body connects to another segment: neck, shoulders, elbows, wrists, fingers, legs, knees, ankles, and toes. Movement of these parts involves rotating clockwise and counterclockwise, bending and pulling or pushing slightly.

There is almost nothing one can do to decrease the benefits of a massage. Notice we said almost. Holistic body and massage therapists note that varying hand motions are important in order to prevent tedium. Likewise, a caring attitude assures that the healing energies of the therapist are accentuated in the needed area. Without these two very important assets, therapy can become ineffectual. As we discuss a few of the therapies available to consumers in the next section, please notice that even though each method is considered by its practitioners as holistic, many exclude one or more of the important elements of holism contained in other healing systems discussed in this book.

Type of Healing Method

Even though there are many types of massage or body therapy, we are only going to familiarize you with Rolfing, Reichian therapy, shiatsu, polarity, and reflexology, since they are the most popular methods. The major difference between them is the emphasis of their technique and their application to the whole person. Many also accentuate structural factors, whereas others stress emotional factors.

Rolfing, the first step we will discuss, is also known as *Structural Integration* (Feitis, 1978; Rolf, 1977). This is a method of structural realignment of the body segments so that they are vertically aligned. Its hand movements encompass deep massage with knuckles, elbows, finger pressure, rolling, and manipulation and are used to reshape physical posture. Each body is considered individual in structure, and vertical balance is accomplished according to weight and maladjustment. Rolfing is completed through ten one-hour sessions designed to lengthen, straighten, and balance the body in relation to the pull of gravity.

Practitioners begin with surface skin and muscles and progress to deep muscles, nerves, and connective tissues. By using their hands, Rolfers force the parts of the body to move into vertical position. Rolfers report that their clients do feel some pain during sessions because pressure has been released, and soreness is felt afterward until the body becomes reacclimated to its correct vertical position. The pain experienced while being manipulated often releases emotional energies that have been held internally. Consequently emotional reactions are also associated with Rolfing.

According to Ida Rolf, Ph.D., founder of the method, a structurally balanced body should be:

1. Knees vertical over the ankles,
2. Hips vertical over the knees,
3. Shoulders vertical over the hips, and
4. Ears vertical over the shoulders.

Rolfers are of the opinion that our ideas about "correct posture" work against our body structure. These therapists are not considered to be massage therapists, for their emphasis is upon the restructuring of the whole body so that it projects an outward picture of balance and symmetry. The individual, as a result of Rolfing, gains greater energy use from the muscular system.

There is some evidence to support the Rolf system of Structural Integration. Dr. Valerie Hunt and Dr. J. Silverman have completed some research on the aftereffects of Rolfing. Silverman reports that changes often associated with emotional release take place biochemically, and Hunt found that more efficient use is made of muscular energy after the Rolfing process. Additionally, these researchers found that reflexive responses are polished rather than jerky, which allows energy to be conserved (Hunt, 1977; Silverman et al., 1973). The body, then, is balanced, thereby assuring the client of skillful physical actions and an even flow of energy. Because the body is made up of four large segments (head, thorax, pelvis, and legs), according to these practitioners, it can be altered. Rolfers change these body segments so that the connecting portions move freely and subtly. Vertically aligned, the energy received from the force of gravity supports the body, whereas when one is malaligned, the energy is misplaced.

Rolfers neither consider themselves therapists, nor do they consider their method a cure for dis-eases. They merely teach one how to increase functioning and skillfulness. The therapist, Rolfers espouse, is gravity. Rolfers point out that the energy within gravity is vertical, and when one is vertically sound, gravity passes through the body and enhances its energy flow. Improper postural structure decreases and/or misdirects the natural flow of gravitational energy into the body. The energy associated with gravity has two major purposes: to help support the body and to aid individual transformation of energy for use. A body that is not vertically aligned cannot properly make use of gravity as a functioning integrator. Gravity could, instead, harm the body. Rolfing's aim is to place the body segments into an order that is balanced and energized so that the individual is able to convert gravity's energy into his/her own.

As with most practitioners in the holistic field, Rolfers affirm that outward appearance and/or posture are clues to inner states. By organizing the basic structure of a client, Rolfers feel that physical and emotional potentials are expanded. One outwardly represents symmetry while inwardly balancing the natural energies of the body (Rolfing's inclusion of gravitational energy reminds us of the Native American healer who dances barefoot to exchange positive and negative energies with Mother Earth). As astute observers, Rolfers are able to point out energy-rejecting habits and stances. Furthermore, they instruct one about the best possible means for changing energy-reducing customs.

Reichian therapy is much more complicated. Invented by Wilhelm Reich, a protégé of Freud who was later jailed because of a misconception about his method, bioenergetic therapy encompasses mental-physical relationships with dis-ease. Reich felt that life (orgone) energy flowed freely throughout the body. Emotional conflicts, fear, anger, sadness, neurosis, repressed feelings, and sexual inhibitions were seen as sources of physical dis-ease. Fear and emotional resistance caused "muscular" and "character" "armoring" to take place in the body. With this as his basis, Reich added two techniques to psychotherapy: *Reichian body therapy* and *character analysis*.

According to Reich, the individual is good. "Evil" emerged from inhibiting natural feelings toward love. These emotional inhibitions were also attached to the individual's need to act. However, if one did not react to his or her natural feelings, armoring took place. Suppressed emotions and actions built up until one adopted a character of defensiveness against the natural flow of energy generated from feelings. Reich reasoned that since the body reacts by contracting to repressed stress, releasing the restraints with body therapy would likely allow therapists to examine and dissolve the cause of armoring.

Again, practitioners are provided clues to one's character by observing an individual's "body language": walk, expression, posture, voice, outward display of emotions, and so forth. Therapists begin character analysis by taking one trait and having the client express that trait. For instance, if you are hostile, a therapist would urge you to demonstrate that feeling, hoping to make you consciously aware of its effects. Body therapy, on the other hand, employs many techniques to dissolve the constricted muscular tensions created by inhibitions. In body therapy practitioners begin with the most obviously tense portions of the body and move to the deeper ones. Thus, character analysis and body therapy became the tools of Reichian therapy (Hoff, 1978; Lowen, 1975; Reich, 1973, 1976).

According to these practitioners, individual clients may not be aware of the body's characteristic expressions visible to others. Many become conditioned to "bouncing back" or "putting up a front" in order to protect themselves from being truthful or being hurt. Bioenergetic therapy seeks to relinquish these feelings by combining deep massage, regulation of breath and psychotherapy. Therapists report that Reichian therapy is often emotionally and physically painful for clients. The deep emotional conflicts associated with an individual's character usually evoke emotional convulsions when released. Likewise, methods employed in body therapy can cause physical pain when the repressed energy is freed. However, when the person regains his or her balance and the life energy is once again flowing freely, he or she is able to approach the world in a less defensive and more loving manner. Practitioners of Reichian therapy must be skilled psychiatrists or psychologists because of the mental and physical demands required to undertake this complicated method.

As we explained earlier, the use of Reichian body work allows underlying emotional restraints to emerge. Therapists believe that energy transfers itself in positive, creative forms rather than through negative, deleterious ones. The client must relearn his or her "character." Therapists teach their clients to seek growth and loving interrelationships that are supportive. In many cases, they assert, learning how one "really feels" about self, others, and the world at large is a slow process. This is one reason a trained practitioner is crucial. The therapy is limited without the use of body work, character analysis, and a feeling for the individual as whole.

Another type of therapy is known as *reflexology*, or *zone therapy*. Reflexology is similar to acupuncture in that certain points or energy zones are located on the hands and feet and are linked to different body organs and glands. Reflexologists tell us that points are associated with nerve endings within the hand or foot. Through these points, the reflexologist can adjust the energy flow within the body. Therapists relax and stimulate nerve endings, which induce the same in glands and organs. Reflex points are linked to glands and organs by way of meridians. Massaging one or more points on the hands and/or feet releases the energy blockage in correlated parts of the body, thereby harmonizing or balancing the energy flow throughout the entire system. Practitioners of zone therapy do not regard themselves as healers. Rather, they aid the body in healing itself by enabling the client to "let go" of the energy linked to dis-ease. There is no diagnosis, prescription, or treatment of specific dis-eases (Devaki, 1977).

Reflexologists are of the belief that stresses encountered in daily life create imbalances in the body. These imbalances usually manifest themselves in symptoms of dis-ease. Incorrect assimilation of foods, stress, and social pressures display themselves as energy blockages, causing calcium crystals or small granules and nodules on the feet and/or hands. Reflexologists break down these deposits and open up energy passages to glands and organs. The areas where deposits are found are handled carefully. Practitioners explain that they return to these areas throughout treatment so that the block is dissipated slowly and without pain. Whereas Reichian therapy asserts that the pain associated with energy release is beneficial, reflexologists feel that pain can create further body stress. Unlike the other body therapies we discuss, practitioners of reflexology primarily make use of their thumbs to release energy barriers.

Breath control is often employed to direct concentration to the area being massaged. Therapists encourage clients to breathe deeply and/or ask that they coordinate breath with the practitioner's. Additionally, some practitioners request that clients employ visualization during the massage and picture the energy moving freely through the body. For example, one may visualize the breath giving energy and/or dissipating blockages. Reflexologists explain that breath control and visualization enhance zone therapy by enabling the client to totally relax. This further assures that the vital force is set forth in an unconstrained manner.

Practitioners apply pressure and/or massage specific areas on hands or feet. For example, the ball of the foot is massaged for stomach regulation and pressure is applied to the ends of the toes to manage sinus areas. One entire foot is completed before moving to the other. It is common to feel tired after reflexology massage. Therapists attribute this to the fact that toxins within the body have been liberated so that the body can eliminate them. Some practitioners suggest that clients eat lightly the day after massage in order to enable the body to carry out its excretory processes with greater ease. According to one therapist, resuming the same routine and consuming one's normal food requirements can prevent the body from eliminating the poisons released during reflexology.

A Japanese massage termed *shiatsu* combines sustained pressure and healing concentration into a healing massage therapy. Shiatsu is a deriviation of acupuncture and Western massage methods that makes use of thumbs and fingers during the massage. Practitioners seek to balance the vital energies by massaging yin and yang points located along meridians. According to Shiatsu therapists, the massage is performed perpendicular to the body, providing deeper penetration than either Western methods or acupuncture. Practitioners move along meridians applying continued pressure to subdue the nerves. The treatment, then, is opposite in its effects on the physical body from reflexology and Reichian therapy. Rather than augmenting and exciting bodily functions, Shiatsu decreases and relaxes these functions by focusing on the parasympathetic nervous system (Blate, 1976; Schultz, 1978; Warren, 1976).

Managing a stable pressure is crucial in this school of massage. Therefore, the practitioner's body weight is balanced so that his or her hands and fingers remain steady. Energy imbalances are detected while receiving the massage and the therapist acts as a transfer vehicle by redistributing energy or replacing negative with positive energy. This massage method, they assert, affects the deep organ's systems to initiate the self-healing or balancing processes of the body. Practitioners point out that energy imbalances can be felt and, in some cases, seen by the fingers. The therapist must act as a "ground," meaning that he or she must not only be in a proper position but that the therapist's mind must be totally centered upon the receiver. The shiatsu practitioner must, according to most therapists, maintain an empathetic, egoless mind in order to give the receiver shiatsu massage.

Therapists engage the receiver in spiritual concentration so that both practitioner and client are concentrating thoughts in the corresponding area of treatment. A spiritual bond is constructed between healer and healee in order to contact the healing energies within the body. Some therapists request that clients visualize an energy exchange between them, focusing upon a give-and-take relationship between body and vital energy. Additionally, since shiatsu is very relaxing to the body and mind, therapists point out it is easier for clients to "let go" of dis-ease. In this respect, shiatsu is very much like meditation.

The combination of yin and yang pressure and massage along meridians represents a spiritual-physical union that restores what is called a flexible "equilibrium" to the receiver. The healee is then able to initiate self-healing processes previously subdued. Therapists say that shiatsu is an excellent preventive massage, since it encourages one to totally relax the body and mind, which, in turn, allows the natural processes inherent in the body to readjust themselves. They further relate that imbalances and/or the onset of dis-ease is more easily detected by those who practice shiatsu on a regular basis. For this reason these practitioners claim to "treat and diagnose" simultaneously, which may cause legal problems in the future for this method.

Polarity therapy partially extends the other therapies because it projects a system of health maintenance. Polarity therapy assembles vital energy, diet, positive thinking, manipulation, and exercise. The method is integrated into a client's life-style in order to strengthen and balance mental, physical, and emotional factors. Polarity therapists also focus on energy fields as the nucleus of well-being (Pannetier, 1978). Polarity teachers emphasize that one must build health slowly and steadily by examining unhealthy practices and adding ones that accentuate balance. According to this body therapy, in order to prevent dis-ease one must make use of exterior and interior means to balance the flow of vital energy, thereby maintaining health.

Polarity therapy, then, is also based on energy channels that run from head to toe and are connected to organs and glands. As observed in nature, energy is positive, negative, or neutral. When energy is flowing freely and is balanced, a polarity exists. Energy imbalance creates unhealthy conditions in the organs and glands that are linked to the energy channels. Practitioners assert that they teach clients how to assume responsibility for sustaining energy balance by building self-confidence and integrating health methods into their lives. Exercise instruction is centralized around yoga, posture, movement, and stretching. As in acupuncture, chiropractic, and other holistic methods, clients are taught that posture is important in order to increase vital energy flow. Therefore, maintaining postural alignment is a key factor in polarity exercise programs so that impediments to vital energy flow do not occur.

This is one method that includes dietary education within its framework. Many holistic methods in this book emphasize the significance of cleansing and purifying the body, and polarity is no exception. Practitioners point out that this process is essential to ridding body toxins and building an internal environment that counteracts dis-ease. Polarity therapists concentrate their nutritional education on fresh fruits and vegetables. Natural foods and water consumption are also included in polarity's dietary instruction for clients. These therapists point out that emotional states play a crucial role in the digestion and assimilation of foods. Even though polarity therapy offers some kind of nutritional counseling of its clients (coupled with various exercise methods), the idea that a nutritionally sound body is created only with fresh fruits and vegetables, natural foods, increased consumption of water, and emotional calm while eating may be challenged by some nutritionalists as this therapy gains in popularity.

Since polarity therapists believe that realities are created by individual and group beliefs, practitioners in this field place great value on positive attitudes. Clients are encouraged to improve the self—not only to develop self-confidence but also to learn the unlimited nature of his or her being. Instructors teach clients that growth of the self is a value that promotes well-being. When one inhibits his or her potentials, the innate qualities present within are also hindered, which is similar to Reichian beliefs. According to popularity therapists, individual growth is a natural occurrence. They advise the client to strive for a positive outlook and take steps toward maintaining health and well-being.

After examining the most popular massage and body therapies available to consumers, we conclude that most of them are natural because of their philosophical assumptions and methods of health maintenance that they practice. However, Reichian therapies may pre-scribe drugs due to the fact that most of them are practicing psychia-trists who are licensed to do so. Very few of the massage or body therapies include all the holistic qualities needed to be considered holistic practices, but all incorporate the body-mind relationship to dis-ease, self-regulating processes of the body and energy channels, as well as individual action toward well-being. Concern for total well-being is a responsibility that each consumer must undertake.

Description of Healing Method

Throughout this chapter we discuss hand and finger movement, balanc-ing, exercise strategies, and beliefs upon which massage and body therapies are based to promote well-being. In this section we will try to summarize the massage techniques by presenting a procedure often followed by holistic therapies. We do not by any means suggest that all massages are performed in this way, for as you can see by reading this chapter, many types of therapies exist. We simply want to paint a picture of smooth movement and consistency so that you are able to judge the quality of a massage.

Massages begin by having the receiver lie on his or her stomach. Any private areas are covered if nudity seems to inhibit total relaxation of the client. A pillow is often placed under the head and ankles for comfort and one is asked to relax. In many cases, deep breathing exercises will be employed to increase ease before initiating the mas-sage. Practitioners explain that the receiver is not to help in the massage and if at any time he or she helps, the therapist reminds the client to relax. During this time, one is in a warm room to ensure comfort, since the lubrication makes the body more sensitive to cold. The initial personal contact made between the therapist and receiver is not released until the massage is complete. In order to simplify the massage procedure, we have listed the process somewhat loosely in the following box. Remember also that passive exercise methods should be included.

The Massage Procedure

With lubricated hands, the therapist begins on the back of both arms, moving down to the hands, moving up to the neck, moving down to the shoulders, spine, and buttocks, moving to the back of the legs and completing the back of the receiver with the feet. The same motions are then repeated on the front of the receiver.

Diseases Treated

Remember that most massage and body therapists do not diagnose or treat dis-ease. Instead, they provide relief and/or balance so that the life energies flow unobstructed throughout the body. Massage and body therapies have been useful, then, in furnishing relief, promoting efficiency, and preserving well-being in the following dis-eases: strengthening muscles in multiple sclerosis, restoring movement in paralysis, toning muscles, inhibiting degenerative dis-eases, increasing glandular functioning, preventing nervous disorders, releasing toxins, increasing assimilation, breaking up fatty tissues, stimulating skin functions; and relieving pain, spasms, backaches, tendonitis, sinus problems, headaches, stress, kidney conditions, polio, ulcers, coronary problems, postural defects, fractures, numbness, constipation, arthritis, rheumatism, strains, sprains, cerebral palsy, prostitis, circulation conditions, respiratory congestion, swellings, neuralgia, asthma, immovable joints, stiffness, emotional conflicts, and gastrointestinal conditions.

Duration of Treatment

Rolfing is the only method that specifies its length (see "Type of Healing Method"). Reichian therapy is much more involved. Practitioners often work with clients as long as it takes to analyze the underlying causes of emotional-physical armoring. This method is much like attending analysis sessions. Therefore, release from treatment is dependent upon the therapist's judgment of a cure.

Reflexologists often only administer one treatment and subsequent therapy is left to the client. Shiatsu therapists diagnose and treat dis-ease until the healing process is initiated in the patron. Commonly, this takes only one visit. Polarity therapy teaches health maintenance on a daily basis. In this case, nutrition, positive thinking, massage, manipulation, and yoga are part of a chosen life-style.

Cost Range

Because there are so many separate methods of body therapy, the cost range varies considerably. Reflexologists, shiatsu practitioners, and some massage therapists will provide emergency services and have given their services free of charge.

General massage—sometimes free, but usually $8–$35 per session
Rolfing (10-week session)—donation to $225
Polarity—$20–$30 per session
Shiatsu—free to $30 per session
Reichian therapy—$50–$125 per session
Reflexology—free to $20 per session

Personal Responsibilities

The major concern here is the consumer's realization that those methods that include massage and body therapy are not employed as cures. Although therapists engage in one of the oldest forms of folk medicine, most do not diagnose or treat specific dis-eases. Their overall intention is to exercise tissues, muscles, and nerves as well as removing energy barriers so that the individual can initiate the healing process. Any therapist in this field who claims that he or she can cure dis-ease with his or her particular method is not legitimate.

Numerous divisions within this field make it increasingly difficult to judge which school of thought is best suited to your needs. Hopefully we have provided you with a summary complete enough to spur interest in one of them. Go with the one you like best, for it will be the one that will furnish the most beneficial results. As a prelude, find out if the practitioner is trained and in what type of therapies. Base your final decision upon the quality of the massage or body therapy and the method's intent to educate in order to prevent future imbalance. In addition, check to see if your chosen therapy is employed as a health maintenance measure.

What if you get there, they tell you to remove your clothes, and you do not want to be nude? There are alternatives. Leave on your underwear, go to the table, and assume that the therapist "takes the hint," or tell him or her immediately that nudity will make you uncomfortable. Remember that many people express the same misgivings. Therapists often have gowns or towel robes for use by their clients that are intended to ease this conflict.

Perhaps the most difficult part of the massage for the receiver is to remain completely relaxed. It is quite natural to "help" a practitioner raise an arm or rotate a toe. He or she is to do all the "physical work" for your body. Total abatement allows those tense areas to receive the attention they have long needed. Total relaxation will also facilitate emotional release and free-flowing energy. Emotional release enhances personal well-being, so be aware in advance that any relinquishment of physical or emotional feeling will be accepted by the therapist.

Massage and body therapy is, above all, a health maintenance system that has considerable potential for home implementation. Chronic dis-eases associated with incorrect posture, such as low back pain and headaches, may be prevented by the regular inclusion of one of these therapies. Dietary habits are also important to a healthy body, a clear mind, and a free spirit. As you find yourself assuming responsibility for diet and exercise, an improved self-concept emerges to complete the exchange between spirit, mind, and body and the expansion of your own healing potentials. These are aspects of all holistic methods and often are the hardest for consumers to follow.

Informational Organizations

American Massage and Therapy Association, Inc.
152 West Wisconsin Avenue
Milwaukee, WI 53203

The Alliance of Students and Practitioners of
Medical Massage and Related Therapies
c/o The Swedish Institute
875 Avenue of the Americas
New York, NY 10001

Shiatsu Therapy Center
924 29th Street
Sacramento, CA 95816

Rolf Institute
PO Box 1868
Boulder, CO 80302

Pierre Pannetier Polarity Center
401 North Glassell Street
Orange, CA 92666

Consistencies

1. Practitioners emphasize that the ability to heal resides within the receiver. They merely "clear the channels" so that the process can begin.

2. Incorporation of massage or body therapy is considered an integral aspect of continued well-being in the field of holistic medicine. Not only are there several schools of thought, but they are also used by other practitioners—for example, chiropractors.

3. Self-improvement, self-esteem, and positive beliefs are encouraged by most of the therapies we examined. This means that more than the physical aspects of massage or body therapy must be included before one has a complete holistic health routine in any of these disciplines.

4. Observation of a client's walk, gestures, posture, mannerisms, expressions, habits, and so on are clues for body therapists. Shiatsu and Reichian therapists point out the significance of individual character traits in curing and preventing dis-ease. Even though other methods do not diagnose and treat, special attention is given those observable areas of the individual that need the most relief.

5. Just as meditation brings stress reduction to the mind, body therapy achieves similar results through physical therapy. Further, massage has been legitimated by the medical establishment through its use as an adjunct to conventional treatments.

Inconsistencies

1. Not all of the various body therapies available include nutritional considerations, client education, or spiritual applications within their system. We also found that very little counseling is available about the significance of life-style and mental outlook for maintaining well-being. Thus, some of these fields can be viewed as dealing with only one segment of the whole person.

2. Although there has been a small amount of research completed on Rolfing (shiatsu is now under study), other therapies must rely upon case histories to prove the relevance of their methods to the field of holism. Since practitioners of body therapy or massage consider themselves teachers or masters of an art rather than a science, it is only rarely used as a total healing modality. This may change as more research is published. Usually, from the consumer's viewpoint, these therapies are associated with gyms and health spas. The art of massage is not utilized as a *healing* modality in health spas and gyms.

3. It is obvious from some of the contradictions between various therapies, such as shiatsu and reflexology, that massage, whether holistic or not, possesses internal inconsistencies.

Sources to Read

Bergson, Anika, and **Tuchack, V.** *Zone Therapy.* New York: Pinnacle, 1974.

Blate, Michael. *The G-Jo Handbook.* Davie, FL: Talkynor Books, 1976.

Carter, Mildred. *Helping Yourself with Foot Reflexology.* West Nyack, NY: Parker Publishing Co., 1969.

Chan, Pedro. *Finger Acupressure.* Alhambra, CA: Chan's Books, 1975.

Cyriax, James. *Treatment by Manipulation, Massage and Injection.* Baltimore: Williams and Wilkins, 1971.

Devaki, Berkson. *The Foot Book: Healing With the Integrated Treatment of Foot Reflexology.* New York: Funk and Wagnalls, 1977.

Downing, George. *Massage and Meditation.* New York: Random House, 1974.

———. *The Massage Book.* New York and Berkeley, CA: Random House and The Bookworks, 1972.

Feitis, Rosemary. *Ida Rolf Talks About Rolfing and Physical Reality.* New York: Harper and Row, 1978.

Hofer, Jack. *Total Massage.* New York: Grosset and Dunlap, 1976.

Hoff, Richard. "Overview of Reichian Therapy," *Holistic Health Handbook.* Edward Bauman, et al. Berkeley: And/Or Press, 1978.

Hunt, Valerie V., and **Massey, W.** "Electromygraphic Evaluation of Structural Integration Techniques," *Psychoenergetic Systems*, no. 2 (1977), pp. 199–210.

Irwin, Yukiko, and **Wagenvoord, J.** *Shiatsu: Japanese Finger Pressure for Energy.* Philadelphia: Lippincott, 1976.

Jackson, Richard. *Holistic Massage.* New York: Drake, 1977.

Janov, Arthur. *Prisoners of Pain.* New York: Doubleday, 1980.

Johnson, Don. *The Protean Body: A Rolfer's View of Human Flexibility.* New York: Harper-Colophon, 1977.

Kaye, Anna, and **Matchan, D. C.** *Mirror of the Body.* San Francisco: Strawberry Hill, 1978.

Kellogg, John Harvey. *The Art of Massage.* Mokelumne Hill, CA: Health Research, 1929.

Kloss, Jethro. *Back to Eden.* Santa Barbara, CA: Woodbridge Press, 1975.

deLangre, Jacques. *First Book of Do-In.* Wethersfield, CT: Omangod, 1973.

———. *Second Book of Do-In.* Magalia, CA: Happiness Press, 1974.

Lowen, Alexander. *Bioenergetics.* New York: Viking Press, 1975.

Masunaga, Shizuto. *Zen Shiatsu.* San Francisco: Japan Publications, 1977.

Miller, Roberta. *Psychic Massage.* New York: Harper and Row, 1975.

Namikoski, Tokujiro. *Shiatsu.* San Francisco: Japan Publications, 1974.

———. *Shiatsu Therapy: Its Theory and Practice.* San Francisco: Japan Publications, 1974.

Ohashi, Wataru. *Do It Yourself Shiatsu.* New York: Dutton, 1976.

Pannetier, Pierre. "Polarity Therapy," *Wholistic Dimensions in Healing.* Leslie J. Kaslof, Garden City, NY: Doubleday, 1978.

———. *Health Building.* Orange, CA: Pannetier, 1978.

Reich, Wilhelm. *The Discovery of the Orgone: The Function of the Orgasm.* New York: Noonday, 1971.

———. *Cancer Biopathy.* New York: Farrar, Straus and Giroux, 1973.

———. *Character Analysis.* New York: Simon and Schuster, 1972.

Reilly, Dr. Harold J., and **Brod, R.** *The Edgar Cayce Handbook for Health through Drugless Therapy.* New York: Jove Publications, 1975.

Rolf, Ida P. *Rolfing: The Integration of the Human Structure.* Santa Monica, CA: Dennis-Landman, 1977.

Schultz, Barbara L. "New Age Shiatsu," *Holistic Health Handbook.* Edward Bauman, et al., Berkeley, CA: And/Or Press, 1978.

Serizawa, Katsusuke. *Massage: The Oriental Method.* Elmsford, NY: Japan Publications, 1972.

Silverman, J., et al. "Stress, Stimulus Intensity Control and the Structural Integration Technique," *Confinia Psychiatrica,* 1973, pp. 201–219.

Stone, Randolph. *Energy: The Vital Polarity in the Healing Art.* Oregon, CA: Polarity Therapy, 1948.

———. *Polarity Therapy and Its Tribune Function.* Orange, CA: Polarity Therapy, 1949.

———. *Vitality Balance.* Orange, CA: Polarity Therapy, n.d..

Tappan, Frances M. *Healing Massage Techniques: A Study of Eastern and Western Methods.* Reston, VA: Reston Publishing Co., 1978.

Warren, Frank. *Freedom from Pain through Acupressure.* New York: Wentworth, 1976.

Weinberg, Robert S. and **Hunt, V. V.** "Effects of Structural Integration on State–Trait Anxiety," *Journal of Clinical Psychology* (35) 2, April 1979: pp. 319–322.

13

DREAM THERAPY

Definition

Dreams are symbolic pictures. They represent how one views oneself, one's relationships with others, and the world at a particular point in time. The symbols are created by the dreamer so that he or she can learn from and relate to dreams. They are not random, evil, animalistic drives contained within all people. Instead, they provide insights into feelings, beliefs, and actions. It is for this reason that dreaming has been employed by holistic practitioners.

Dreams, then, give one the opportunity to perceive "another" self, to study the interactions performed on the dream stage, and to learn "extra information" for application in the waking world. As a result, healing problems can be encountered and, in some cases, resolved in the dream world.

Garfield (1979) points out that symbols of health and dis-ease are often portrayed in dreams in order to warn us of physical problems. In

other words, dreaming "offers us unique opportunities for early awareness of our physical as well as our emotional conditions and needs. We
must, first of all, learn to read the symbols of our dreams that present
messages portraying current physical conditions."

Dream therapy is primarily employed by psychologists, dream
groups, or as a complementary modality within acupuncture, meditation, Native American healing, and homoeopathy. Currently, dream
therapy is not a separate healing method. As with music (see Chapter
14), it has been developed for use with behavioral and mental problems.

According to dream specialists, two major misconceptions about
dreaming have kept many people from exploring them. One of these is
that dreams are evil because they speak about the hidden "animalistic"
or "evil" instincts within man. The other mistake is that dreams are a
form of hallucination and/or a sign denoting mental illness. Holistic
dreamers feel that Freud is primarily responsible for society's belief that
dreams are untamed, whereas modern psychiatrists and psychologists
are responsible for the belief that they are hallucinations. Today many
psychiatrists and psychologists have retracted their original generalizations attributed to dreams and have given them a place among techniques for gaining insight into individual eccentricities.

Some people we have interviewed do not believe they dream;
however, everyone dreams. Dreams are a necessary product of consciousness that allows for problem solving, dealing with interactions
with others, production of creative products, personal growth, and any
number of actions that take place in the nonphysical realm of sleep.
Additionally, dreams enable one to explore the unknown self, uncover-
ing suppressed potentials or deficits. Accordingly, holistic dream
therapists believe that the exploration of dreams can produce a need to
create harmony within the dreamer who acknowledges unbalanced
and/or unfulfilled aspects of spirit, mind, emotion, and body.

Symbols in dreams are objects, states of emotion in characters,
places, settings, plots, environments surrounding the dream, animals,
and specific characters themselves. Religious symbols such as crosses,
natural symbols such as sunlight, comments that are remembered, or
colors—are all open to interpretation. These symbols, it is supposed, are
a form of inner guidance that allows for the attainment of smooth interaction between spirit, mind, emotion, and body. Symbols direct the
dreamer's attention to deficits, excesses, or potentials that manifest
themselves in waking life.

In most dreams, the dreamer plays every role. To find the meaning
behind a dream picture, one must use imagination and elaboration.
There are a number of ways to accomplish this. One of the easiest is to
view the dream as a subjective picture of life. "Does the picture represent any truth in waking life?" "What does it tell me about the feelings

and actions of myself?" Another method suggested by Dr. Gayle Delany, a dream psychologist, is to view the dream as someone from another planet would see it. This, of course, is a more objective way of analyzing a dream.

Dreams are also translated through association. A dreamer composes a brief sketch that lists the actors, objects, settings, or words to try and associate meanings with symbols. Often, the "correct" association is the first one that comes to mind. The following dream yielded much insight through association for a dreamer that we interviewed:

> I dreamed I was a slave. The master of the slaves was telling me and three others to keep working. We wanted to rest and eat, but he beat us into line with his whip.

In this dream the following list of symbols and associations was made by the dreamer:

> slave master—dominated by work, he is mean and cruel; he carried a whip
> slaves—wanted freedom, rest, food, and other activities
> rest—more play activities needed in life, need rest to work more efficiently
> food—he or she was not eating enough
> work—all the slave master thought about; the slaves were doing all the labor

Although this is a relatively simple association, it is quite easy to understand the method.

It is easy to see how a specific dream like this can affect the physical well-being of the dreamer. "Workaholics" are the victims of chronic dis-eases caused by overindulgence in long, arduous hours of work. If the dreamer had not "listened" to the dream, it is possible that she might have driven herself to physical dis-ease.

Establishing a dream group may be very helpful in sorting out and gaining insight into a number of different types of dreams. Dream groups supply objective reactions to dreams. In many cases, the meanings of symbols may not be procured very easily by the dreamer. Group members can furnish their individual feelings and thoughts, which are usually quite different from those of the dreamer. It is important that participants in the group do not analyze or interpret a dream, for this must be achieved by the dreamer. A common method of dream cognition carried out in groups is that of the hot seat. Placing two chairs next to each other, the dreamer swaps roles and talks with dream characters and symbols. Symbols may be objects, characters, animals, designs, or natural phenomena such as trees. Positions in the chairs are changed in order to make the transition from one character to the other. The chair thereby facilitates role change for the dreamer. Group members question the symbols in order to shed light on their meaning. A significant point here is why one symbol is chosen over another. For example, a dream symbol may be a swamp instead of a grassy field. Why did the dreamer choose this symbol?

Topdog, underdog is still another technique for analyzing the meanings and symbols of dreams. One dream symbol takes the dominant role while the other takes the subordinate role. Members question both roles to find out why one is dominating the other. This technique is especially useful in dreams because the dreamer is able to resolve the conflicts existing between interrelated, contrasting selves.

Thus far we have discussed how dreams explicitly relate to waking life. In our example the dream represents the dreamer's personal conflicts that could cause future physical problems. According to dream therapists, dream study can prevent mental conflicts from gaining control of physical weaknesses in that once the dreamer is made aware of a problem, it is easier to find a solution. This process allows the dreamer to become aware and take control of events that may hinder his or her well-being.

There are a number of questions that throw light on the meanings of symbols and the plots of dreams. A partial list of these follows. Other questions, more appropriate for your dream perhaps, can also be asked so that you can gain the greatest insight into your dream scenes. These are intended just to give you an idea of the questioning process that is needed to interpret individual dreams and symbols.

1. Does the dream relate to waking life in any way?
2. Does the dream contain any objective truth?
3. Does the dream speak directly to me? What did it say?
4. Does the dream offer creative potentials?
5. Does the dream point out physical problems? Corrections?
6. Do the characters reflect parts of my personality?
7. Do the dream symbols talk of my feelings? Which ones? About what?
8. Do the dream symbols talk about how I see my world? In what manner?
9. Do the dreams present solutions to problems?
10. What symbols are used? Why are those particular symbols used? What is their meaning?
11. Do series of dreams/symbols relate to each other?
12. Does the dream picture any conflicts? What are they?
13. Does the dream point out destructive impulses? Such as?
14. What negative factors are contained in the dream? Positive ones?

Erich Fromm (1951) has called the language of dreams a "symbolic" one. The meanings of dream symbols can change. Sometimes they can change meanings with each dream. There are many excellent sources that report symbolic meanings for specific symbols, and in some cases, specific types of dreams—such as flying dreams, dreams of houses, or dreams of animals—reveal certain themes. It is best, however, to derive the personal significance for each dream symbol rather than interpreting its scope as a book would. Each dream sequence is highly individualized and its meaning may be entirely different for one dreamer than for another.

There are many types of dreams. Nightmares occur to most everyone and are usually recurring. Nightmares and/or recurring dreams are pointing out something of importance to the dreamer. The dream and its characters and plots, no matter how horrible, are created by the dreamer and can therefore be destroyed by the dreamer. Ann Faraday suggests repeating the phrase "You have no power over me" to monsters and evil villains in nightmares. Although many of us have experienced nightmares, other types of dreams are just as common. Some other kinds of dreams and examples of each are as follows (Faraday, 1973; Garfield, 1974; Sechrist, 1968):

Reminder dreams—A member of our dream group had been looking for a brownie recipe for three months, but she couldn't find it. She had the following dream: "I opened my Christmas cooking folder and the recipe was inside."

Clairvoyant dreams—This dream came from a group member who lived across the country from his family: "There is a green VW going down a road too fast. It comes to a crossroad and cannot stop. It sideswipes another car and rolls into a ditch." He called home two days later and was told that his brother had totaled his new green VW. The wreck had happened while he slept. Fortunately, no one was hurt.

Precognitive dreams—Elsie Sechrist (1968) reports that "President Abraham Lincoln repeatedly dreamed of looking into a mirror opposite his bed. He saw two images of himself, one a reflection of himself in good health, the other a ghost."

Warning dreams—A member of our dream group told of this dream: "I was rafting down the Colorado River. The raft hit a large rock. All I saw after that was a torn-up raft." He didn't take the rafting trip as he had planned. He heard later that the crew had hit a rock, lost all their supplies, and were rescued by an emergency team.

Flying and falling dreams—These dreams are common to all of us. A floating sensation is associated with flying as is the feeling of the wind. Falling dreams often point out a fear in the dream itself. These disappear if the fear is faced either in the dream state or in waking reality.

Dreamlets—Dreamlets occur before one falls to sleep. They are images, colors, schemes, or thoughts acted upon, and often review the day. They are not usually significant.

The "mystery" surrounding the dream state resides in lucid and creative dreaming. These are states in which the dreamer can control, become consciously aware of, and change the dream contents to suit his or her fantasy or taste. Many great inventors and intellectuals are stereotyped as being immersed in their work and absorbed with the outcome of the product. Einstein, Edison, Emerson, and many others reported that sleep was the principal experimental grounds for ideas before they were applied and given "form" in physical life. Creative dreamers, inventers, and poets make use of the dream world for "trying out" conceptions. Adjustments, expansions, and innovations can be verified before the "working model" is created. Thus, creative dreaming has given us some of our most advanced inventions and scientific ideas.

"Lucid" dreaming is somewhat different from creative dreaming. In lucid states the dreamer is aware that he or she is dreaming. Usually one awakens soon after discovering that he or she is dreaming, concluding that "its only a dream." However, it is possible to remain asleep and be consciously aware of a dream. Yogis, Indians, and other ancient dreamers report that it is possible to change the contents of lucid dreams, manipulate, transform, and make use of them in waking life. This technique, of course, takes many years of study and practice.

Studying dream states can be fun and enlightening. This healing modality, while mental, does facilitate other, more physical methods and may become a distinct branch of psychiatry in the near future. Until that time, however, dream study is one measure from which consumers may profit by establishing health and/or acquiring new perceptions into unhealthy actions, emotions, and thoughts. To achieve and/or support health through dreaming, the consumer takes control of a planned health program constructed especially for his or her own needs.

Types of Healing

Healing within dreaming is the activation of positive resources within an individual. Healing evolves when the dreamer, as Garfield (1979) puts it, "confronts and conquers, disease-producing emotional and conflictual states in the dream world." Dream characters, or allies, can be called upon to help defeat dis-ease. As in Native American rituals, where the shaman asks heroes and heroines to aid the healee, these "participants in the dream" offer valuable information about curing disease that is, although unexplained, "known" somewhere within the individual. Well-being is maintained by the use of visualizations of vitality or symbols of health and well-being. Dreams, when employed for healing, are used as catalysts, incubated, or employed after waking as visualizations. Just as hypnotic suggestions implant the idea of health, health states can be included during dreams.

Man has made use of dreaming from the early phases of society.

Ancient healing priests purified the body (through fasting and water therapy) and shrouded one in a white cloth. Then one would be led into a temple for prayer to the gods. Patients were told to ask for visitations, oracles, or dreams to heal and teach them how to live. Often priests would dress as gods or goddesses and "treat" the healee while asleep with "words to live by," natural remedies, or suggestions for better health. Upon waking, healees would speak of gods telling them how to heal themselves. Priests used many methods and became "agents for putting one in contact" with the forces surrounding the healee. The idea of treating all forces—that is, aspects—of an individual was never questioned because it was assumed that all parts equally influenced one's life on earth. Dream therapists today employ many of these same techniques. The aim of ancient priests was to put the healee in contact with himself or herself, thereby providing a pathway to the source of dis-ease (Stone, 1979).

A concept similar to the techniques utilized by healing priests is that of dream incubation, frequently employed as a method of dream therapy. Somewhat like conditioning or programming, the dreamer plans his or her dream. Before sleep, and while drowsy, one visually experiences thoughts or activities associated with health and the out- come these will have in waking life. For an arthritic person such a visualization may be playing golf on a hot clear day or playing the piano with nimble fingers. This technique can induce a dream sequence in which the healee participates as a "picture of health." However, it may take more than one try to produce the desired results.

A waking visualization is one way in which the dreamer can merge dream and waking worlds. A dreamer expands the scope of a dream during the day. Time is spent during relaxation, exercise, before nap- ping, while eating, or driving home in traffic in developing the dream from the night before. Dream therapists point out that the use of creative imagination strengthens the "tie" between waking and sleeping realities, replenishing vitality and unity between·both states. According to dream therapists, this method allows the healee to mold his or her own continuity and create a state of well-being.

Thinking in terms that represent the *ideals* of health just before sleeping is another effective technique. One can imagine well-being and this thought can serve as a catalyst for health dreams. Health symbols serve the same purpose. For example, one member of the dream group hung a picture of a man climbing a sheer mountain cliff on his wall. Before sleeping, he looked at the picture and imagined himself climbing that mountain. To this inactive man, the picture and subsequent dreams provided the impetus for learning the skills of mountain climbing as well as adding much needed physical activity to his life-style.

Dream therapy is one method with which a consumer can put holism into practice, judge the effects, and not have to hire a professional. Of course, this includes taking responsibility for healthy eating and exercise, too. In most cases, the consumer has an advantage over professionals because pictures and interpretations come from the dreamer. Professionals ask the same questions about dreams that you can ask yourself. There are any number of books that are excellent guides to exploration in this field. They usually present concise information on dream therapy, leaving the majority of the book to explain how dreams can be viewed and interpreted.

A great deal of concentration is also needed for lucid dreaming. We have discovered that becoming cognizant in a dream takes an average of three months in order to learn the surroundings, characteristics, and languages of the dream world. But, first one must master basic dream skills described throughout this chapter. Then it is time to expand the dreamer's role in conscious construction of dream reality.

Our research states that many years of study are needed to control dream contents and to make use of dream products in waking life. However, the serious student of dream therapy may not find this to be true. Numerous dreamers have reported that it took a year or a year and a half to become lucid during dreams. It does take longer to maintain enough control to do whatever one wishes (to do) in a lucid state. Choices are made in dreams. If a dreamer decides not to participate in a dream, all he or she has to do is decide on another topic.

Finally, there is a danger of taking dreams too seriously. This usually arises when one is trying too hard to understand the contents of a dream or when dreams seem too insignificant to have meaning. In the first place, all dreams have meaning, even if they are simple meanings. Not all dreams relay "heavy" or "mystical" messages. There are many funny dreams with symbols that are comical. A dream will tell you quite literally that you *need* to make a monkey out of yourself.

Description of Healing Method

According to holistic dream therapists, dreams are healing because they destroy self-indulgent or self-destructive images held by the healee and foster self-confidence and expanded awareness of the world at large. For instance, one may have the belief that he or she is emotionally stable yet dreams may be chaotic, showing the opposite. Dreams offer a water hole in a desert, but, as you know, the pump must be continually primed in order to obtain more water.

Learning to record dreams is the first step in initiating a dream program. The phrase "I shall wake up and write down a dream tonight" repeated three or more times a day and before sleep works to facilitate the process. It usually takes about three or four days to "catch" a dream. If after a week of not recalling dreams, some find it necessary to set an alarm clock to wake up every two hours in order to "train" yourself.

Prepare sleeping quarters for dream recording by adding a notebook and pen to a bedside table. It is more effective to keep all dreams together not only to study them in sequence but also to keep track of them. A tape recorder can be utilized with greater ease if you can afford one. For writing, a small light may be necessary to keep the brightness from waking you fully. Many have found a night light plugged in next to the bed provides enough light to see and not enough to totally awaken them. Record dreams in the present rather than in past tense and first person rather than second (or third).

Upon awakening, *gently* ease up to write or record the dream. Sudden jolts transfer a dreamer's thoughts from the dream to something else. Write down the dream in the order that you remember it most clearly. Many find that the end comes first, with preceding events following the finale. Try to put down your impressions about the dream, plot, setting, characters, feelings, or any associations, especially words or phrases heard, *at that time*. Do not wait until morning to record these "extras," for they may have become mixed with another dream and/or changed in meaning. The entire process takes about ten minutes.

Diseases Treated

Psychosomatic dis-ease, drug dependency, schizophrenia, skin disorders, tumors, neuritis, bursitis, emotional disorders, melancholia, fear, repression, depression, anxiety, alcoholism, tobacco dependency, obesity, and ulcers.

Duration of Treatment

Should you decide to seek help from dream practitioners, visits can be quite lengthy and expensive. Because combined methods of psychotherapy are employed, psychologists and psychiatrists, the primary professionals in this field, tend to spend weeks interpreting dreams. Therapy begins by learning to record dreams. Instruction is also given on how to prepare for interpretation with the therapist. This very basic procedure can take two separate trips with a cost accompanying each visit. The length of therapy itself can take six weeks to a year for simple problems and longer for more complicated dis-eases.

It is more beneficial and less expensive to join a dream group, form a dream group, or work with your dreams alone. Many dream groups are organized by psychologists or interested individuals and meet for an agreed-upon period of time. Often it is difficult to find out about these types of groups, for they rarely advertise in newspapers. Most groups vote on a date and length of time for group meetings. There is no set time, but they usually meet continuously because of the comaraderie that builds up and the valuable insights gained from group meetings. For those of you who live in college areas, dream groups may be easier to locate. Departments of psychology in colleges and universities are aware of most of the professionals in an area leading groups and can give you a name to contact.

Healing is only dealt with minimally in dream therapy. Well-being is the culmination of exploring the inner self through dreams. Dream professionals point out that studying dreams is only supplemental to other therapies that directly affect dis-ease. Practitioners promote the message that dis-ease must begin in the spiritual and mental realms before it shows itself in the physical body. They report that for healing methods to cure, treatment must deal with "other" realms of experience. It is precisely these other levels that dreams represent.

Cost Range

> Professionally organized group—$7–$45
> Psychotherapist—$20–$78 per hour
> Psychologist—free to $60 per hour

Personal Responsibilities

Unless you feel that this chapter has taught you all there is to know about dream therapy, you will want to spend some money buying a book on dreaming. Many such books are included in our resource list at the end of the chapter. Flip through any prospective purchase to see if it offers information on the interpretation of symbols and the application of dream meanings to life. Some excellent works are available for two to five dollars.

Before you begin working with dreams, you will have to accept on faith the fact that all characters, objects, and situations are created by the dreamer. Verification of this is supposed to occur as you work on the meaning of your dreams. "Don't worry. It's only a dream" must not be used as a rationalization to overlook the scope of a dream. You will have to credit *yourself*, not another force or other people, with dream contents. It takes a lot of gumption to "own up" to our inconsistencies, biases, faults, guilts, and actions. The dream artist utilizes dream worlds to change his or her "personal movie" so that it flows exquisitely, personifying the interconnection between spirit, mind, and body.

The Sundance Community distributes a spiritually oriented dream journal. It provides space for writing, activities to experience, and tips for working on dreams. However, a notebook or pad works just as well, although it does not, of course, provide the same type of inspiration. We found that the ordinary diary does not allow for enough room for expansion of dreams on the small, dated pages. Easy access to dreams is another advantage of using a notebook.

The most difficult responsibility for dreamers is taking the time to put a dream's lesson to use while awake. This is the essential element in learning, expanding and gaining from dream artistry. Beginning dreamers are often embarrassed by the incongruities portrayed in dreams and want to deny or avoid them. Remember that holism seeks to integrate and resolve inconsistencies so that general well-being is achieved. Do not, therefore, be afraid to face up to them, since resolution is more important than the specific beliefs.

Holistic dream therapists believe that work on dreams will not be wasted effort. Creative expression, control, personal integrity, adventure, advice, resolutions of conflicts, understanding, self-expression, and enlightenment are some of the "gifts" given to those who have mastered dreaming. It is during lucid dreaming that a special emphasis is placed upon healing by most of the therapists we interviewed. There is a "carry-over" effect, according to dream masters, in which the conquest of dis-ease in the dream state can be carried over to the physical state.

Practitioners who employ dream therapy usually do so as a part of psychotherapy. Be sure to find out how much time will be spent on dreams. If a group is offered, it would be best to join it because the focus will be on dreams alone instead of a full program of psychoanalysis. Strictly speaking, dream therapy does not incorporate nutrition, exercise, and life-style changes as parts of the healing program.

Informational Organizations

Dream Counselors, Inc.
135 Madison Avenue
Albuquerque, NM 87123

Dream Dynamics
25 Sullivan Avenue
Farmingdale, NY 11735

Poseidia Institute
PO Box 180
Virginia Beach, VA 23458

Association for Research and Englightenment
PO Box 595
Virginia Beach, VA 23451

The Sundance Community
PO Box 595
Virginia Beach, VA 23451

Consistencies

1. Dream therapy validates the concept that individuals create dis-ease and well-being. Development of the self, through the study of dreams and changes in beliefs about ease and dis-ease, provides a new conqruency between mind and body that may also be extended to include attitude toward the world at large.

2. While dream therapy does not provide any physical treatment per se, holistic dream therapists emphasize the interrelationship of spirit, mind, and body. This loosely organized field is based upon the assumption that individuals are responsible for their own state of being and can alter these states through the conscious manipulation of their own unconscious mind by mastering their dreams.

3. Dream therapy is one of the most ancient traditions of healing and has been found to exist in almost every classical civilization in one form or another. It was only with the societal belief that mental phenomena were not important that the therapy because lost as an overemphasis upon physical health became important.

4. As an adjunctive therapy, dream analysis is quite similar to meditation and visualization in that the mind is viewed as a major source of well-being. Modern science is just now beginning to rediscover the significance of the mind in all areas of life, especially the healing arts. This is one major assumption of holistic philosophy.

5. Dream therapy assumes that each person is composed of multiple personalities created by the dreamer and expressed in all of the characters in dreams. This assumption emphasizes the multidimensionality of each person, which is a tenet of the holistic philosophy. The interdependence of these personalities with physical, social, and environmental aspects of each individual are an integral part of holistic health.

Inconsistencies

1. Though the philosophy of dream therapy emphasizes the interrelationship of mind and body, it does not offer multidimensional programs of holistic health. The neglect of nutritional counseling, exercise, and changes in life-style from programs in dream therapy implies that it is only an adjunct to other forms of healing and places it in the same category as music therapy, massage, and hydrotherapy.

2. At present, dream therapy is not a fully developed healing modality. This situation has both positive and negative consequences for the consumer. A positive consequence is that many of the dangers of overstandardization are absent, allowing for more individualized treatment by the professional. A negative impact of this situation is that there are more opportunities for frauds and charlatans to develop, since there are no professional mechanisms for establishing and enforcing ethical standards and practices.

3. Psychiatrists and psychologists currently dominate this field. This is important because dream therapy comprises only a small proportion of most programs in psychotherapy, and many consumers are interested in the study of their dreams but reluctant to be stigmatized as "mentally unbalanced."

4. Dream therapy is not for everyone. It is very "self" oriented. Practitioners, far and few between, have not communicated the revelance of dream study to the public. Therefore, there are not much published experimental data on healing, and few are lecture seminars given regarding dream states and healing. Therefore, the field presents a "closed" image.

Sources to Read

Baylis, Janice. *Dream Dynamics and Decoding: An Interpretation Manual.* Sun/Man/Moon Publishing Co.: New York Dover Pictorial Archives Series, 1977.

Brain/Mind Bulletin. Los Angeles: Interface Press, 1978–1982.

Bro, Harmon. *Edgar Cayce on Dreams.* New York: Warner Books, 1968.

Brown, Barbara B. *Supermind: The Ultimate Energy.* New York: Harper and Row, 1980.

Campbell, Jean. *Dreams beyond Dreaming.* Virginia Beach, VA: Donning, 1980.

Castaneda, Carlos. *The Eagle's Gift.* New York: Simon and Schuster, 1981.

——. *The Second Ring of Power.* New York: Simon and Schuster, 1977.

——. *Tale of Power.* New York: Simon and Schuster, 1974.

Crisp, Tony. *Do You Dream: How to Gain Insight into Your Dreams.* New York: Dutton, 1972.

Crum, K. *Art of Inner Listening: Pathway to Creativity.* New York: Family Library, 1975.

DeBecker, Raymond. *The Understanding of Dreams.* New York: Weiser, 1914.

Delaney, Gayle. *Living Your Dreams.* New York: Harper and Row, 1979.

Faraday, Dr. Ann *The Dream Game.* New York: Harper and Row, 1974.

———— *Dream Power.* New York: Berkeley Publishing, 1973.

Fromm, Erich. *The Forgotten Language.* New York: Holt, Reinhart and Winston, 1951.

Garfield, Patricia. *Creative Dreaming.* New York: Simon and Schuster, 1974.

————. "Wholistic Health and Dream Work: Using Dreams to Enhance Health," in *Dimensions in Wholistic Healing*, Herbert A. Otto and James W. Knight, ed. Chicago: Nelson-Hall, 1979.

Harvey, Bill. *Mind Magic*, 3d ed. New York: Irvington Publishers, 1980.

Jung, C. G. *Memories, Dreams, Reflections.* London: Collings, 1963.

Kelsey, Morton. *Dreams: A Way to Listen to God.* New York: Paulist Press, 1978.

Koestler, Authur. *The Act of Creation.* New York: Macmillan, 1964.

MacKenzie, Norman. *Dreams and Dreaming.* London: Aldus Books, 1965.

McClashan, Alan. *Savage and Beautiful Country: The Secret Life of the Mind.* New York: Stonehill, 1976.

McLeester, Dick. *Welcome to the Magic Theatre: A Handbook for Exploring Dreams.* Amherst, MA: Published by author, 1976.

Oswald, Ian. *Sleeping and Waking.* New York: Elsevier, 1962.

Peterson, Marilyn. *Nightlights.* Virginia Beach, VA: ARE Press, 1976.

Rassi, Ernest. *Dreams and the Growth Personality.* New York: Pergamon Press, 1971.

Reed, Henry, ed. *The Sundance Community Dream Journal.* Virginia Beach, VA: ARE Press, biannually.

Regush, June and **Nicholas.** *Dream Words, The Complete Guide to Dreams and Dreaming.* New York: New American Living, 1977.

Roberts, Jane. *The Individual and The Nature of Mass Events.* Englewood Cliffs, NJ: Prentice-Hall, 1981.

————. *The Nature of the Psyche.* Englewood Cliffs, NJ: Prentice-Hall, 1979.

————. *The Unknown Reality, Volume One.* Englewood Cliffs, NJ: Prentice-Hall, 1977.

————. *The Unknown Reality, Volume Two.* Englewood Cliffs, NJ: Prentice-Hall, 1979.

————. *Adventures in Consciousness.* Englewood Cliffs, NJ: Prentice-Hall, 1975.

————. *The Nature of Personal Reality.* Englewood Cliffs, NJ: Prentice-Hall, 1974.

Samuels, Mike and **Nancy.** *Seeing with the Mind's Eye.* New York and Berkeley: Random House, 1975.

Sanford, John A. *Dreams and Healing.* New York: Harper and Row, 1980.

Sechrist, Elsie. *Dream Your Magic Mirror.* New York: Warner Books, 1968.

Seigal, Alan. "Dreams: The Mystery That Heals," in *Holistic Health Handbook*, ed. Edward Bauman et al. Berkeley, CA: And/Or Press, 1978.

Shelly, Violet. *Symbols and the Self.* Virginia Beach, VA: ARE Press, 1976.

Starrett, Barbara. *I Dream in Female.* San Fransisco: Cassandra, 1976.

Stone, Harold. "Wholistic Healing: Historic Base and Short History," in

Dimensions in Wholistic Healing, ed. Herbert A. Otto and James W. Knight. Chicago: Nelson-Hall, 1979.

Ullman, Montague, and **Zimmerman, Nan.** *Working with Dreams.* New York: Delacorte Press, 1980.

Von Gruenbaum, G. E., and **Caillois, Roger.** *The Dream and Human Societies.* Berkeley, CA: University of California Press, 1966.

14

MUSIC THERAPY

Definition

Melodies appear to be both subconscious and conscious representatives of our culture. Sounds do not have to be musical. They can be natural, such as birds and crickets in the early evening, ocean waves lapping on the seashore, or a waterfall roaring onto the rocks below. The repetroire is infinite. We can concede that music permits one to "drift away" or relax. But, sounds have a far greater benefit than has previously been speculated.

Ancient civilizations made use of music in many ways. Chants, nonsensical songs, power songs, and harmonious tones were not only used for healing but also for teaching and creative expression. Pythagoras not only derived the Pythagorean Theorem, he also founded a school of philosophy based upon music and numbers. He believed that music and diet could cleanse body and soul. Hindu and Buddhist priests found that each body held a specific tone, and they made use of tones of healing, restoring physical and mental imbalance, and expanding consciousness.

While researching music therapy, we also came across some evidence that implied that some civilizations specialized in the uses of music. Lawrence Blair (1977) reports similar conclusions. He speaks of societies in Mexico and Peru that cut huge stone by producing sound along "precise harmonic lines" and "resonated them [the stones] into position." With this in mind, is it not feasible that a tone can indeed harmonize a body?

With its universal appeal, we thought music therapy would be a highly developed field. However, its tones are only undercurrents in holism, providing the necessary outreach, relaxation, and expansion as adjuncts to other forms of healing. Alas, music is considered by its experts as most effective on behaviors or disabilities. Professionals only indirectly speak of music's balancing capabilities or of its ability to expand the spirit.

Music can create harmony in the physical structure. It is possible to create balancing tones so that the body re-creates a steady state. When used continuously, one can teach the body to revive the tonal frequency when it is needed. The idea of "harmony" indicates that more than one note is used at the same time. Perhaps the idea of harmony, as explained in other chapters, arose from the concept that more than one tone occurs simultaneously. This might have indicated to ancient healers that a state of harmony must be achieved in more than one manner (that is, spirit, mind, and body) in order to perfect a cure.

Researchers report that sound "connects" with the right hemisphere of the brain. The right side is often associated with intuition, nonverbal meaning, pictures, creativity, and healing, whereas the left side allies itself with words, logic, systems, problem solving, and rational thought (see *Brain Mind Bulletin* for the years 1979 through 1981). Modern societies have, for the most part, concentrated their efforts toward developing the left hemisphere, according to most researchers, for use of its logic and practical knowledge. The left side, then, is dominant, which inhibits assets of the right hemisphere because it has been trained almost too effectively.

Brain research intimates that in order for healing to be initiated by tone, it must connect in the right hemisphere and be made real in the left. Both hemispherical processes, then, play an important role in an outcome or cure. Music practitioners must maneuver clients to expand right-brain ability and exercise left-brain interaction to affect balance or a cure. The goal of music therapy in healing is to find out which musical tones create what bodily reactions and to locate the exact tone that rebalances bodily processes.

Music is considered an "emerging field" within medicine. Currently, most of music's expertise is focused solely on "socially and emotionally maladjusted adolescents and adults, with the mentally retarded or with geriatric patients in hospitals, clinics, day care facilities, community mental health centers, and special agencies" (pamphlet from the National Association for Music Therapy, Inc.). According to this definition, music therapists only have a minute role in the overall healing of dis-ease.

Jennifer Rieger (1980), working with confused and disoriented elderly clients, found that reality orientation with music therapy proved highly significant in aiding order of the world for elderly clients. P. C. Liederman (1967) found that rhythm group therapy contributed to both the psychological and physical well-being of geriatric patients. These therapists suggest that the tonal movement within musical scores and the ease that music generates account for its success. Elderly patients adjust to musical tones by moving in a self-adjusting manner, whereas the music itself provides the cornerstone for communication within the "real" world.

Music therapists working with exceptional children find music to be the ideal link to normality. Experts point out that special persons respond to accomplishment demands when music is incorporated into the individualized educational structure that is constructed for exceptional students (Alley, 1979). Furthermore, because music has furnished self-achievement, self-esteem is gained in that students feel more accepted emotionally and socially than they did before music therapy. Kay Roskan (1979) demonstrated that music therapy is a viable means for improving reading skills and increasing auditory awareness in learning-disabled students.

Other important inroads in music therapy have recently become known. Some of this progress is in the critical area of healing. Asthmatic children whose dis-ease had been supplemented with music therapy displayed a stronger pulmonary function, a reduction of progression, and an extension of emotional benefits. Psychodrama ensembles also allow participants to express a wide variety of human emotions. Musical moods and qualities are given to disturbing dreams through musical roleplaying so that emotional problems stemming from them are resolved (Morena, 1967). Additionally, techniques utilized within music therapy have given the physically disabled and elderly new movement.

As this research explicitly demonstrates, music communicates when other methods fail. If we examine current practices in the field of music therapy, we are able to see that the professionals themselves have contributed to the lack of applicability in the field of healing. Music therapists commonly work as part of a health team in clinics, hospitals, prisons, social health centers, and geriatric centers. They share equally in analysis of problems and plan for the general treatment or education of individual clients. Many are employed in special education programs in public and private institutions, and a few others work alone, receiving clientele from health professionals. Therapy in public and private institutions consists of drawing to music, dancing, exercising, taking the rhythm of others, learning, enjoying the melody, and thereby creating what music makes one feel. In some cases, playing an instrument or using voice are incorporated into institutional programs (Braswell, dileo Maranto, and deCuir, 1979).

Guided imagery will more than likely be music therapy's ticket as a healing procedure. In this method a client uses music to relax deeply. Therapists then examine images, feelings, or symbols that emerge while the client is in this state. This technique is employed by practitioners to understand the subconscious thoughts and feelings of clients and to aid the therapist with insights into the individual. Not only has this method proved viable in communication, but it also provided the client with a basis for self-understanding.

There has also been a relatively small amount of research on the association between learning and music. However, Europeans have utilized music to suggest different beliefs or states of mind. Philipov (1979) states that the suggestopedic method makes use of unconscious activity to aid in the learning experience. While reporting on a Bulgarian experiment that involved teaching foreign languages, she explains that the material is received by audio and visual sensors while one is simultaneously learning the written exercise. Therefore, the lesson is taught both consciously and subconsciously and is communicated to both left and right brain hemispheres. She reports that those receiving instruction in this manner learn faster and retain more material for a longer period of time.

Karin Brydon and William Nugent (1979) performed clinical studies of communication processes between the two hemispheres of the brain. These researchers found that communication and assessment in the right hemisphere of the brain focuses on three major methods: music, metaphor, and visualization. Their findings exemplify the distinction between left and right hemispherical processes and serve to prepare the way for music's entrance into the field of healing.

Consumers making use of music as therapy on a regular basis report that memory is enhanced by applying musical tones to important facts. For example, a businessman explained that he needed to remember a large number of statistical facts and background incidental characteristics. He recorded these over a Chopin sonata in B-flat minor. As the sonata played, the "facts and characteristics" were given different form, making them easier to remember. When the piece was recalled, the businessman "heard" the sonata in his head, and as it progressed, the facts were released from his memory.

Most avid music listeners and artists report that time and space are nonexistent when concentration on the music is total. Along with others, they feel that this is directly related to the expansion of conscious awareness. One who is unaware of time and space has opened a new area in the psyche, making room for other experiences. Meditators agree by saying that mantras and chants initiate similar reactions. The healing abilities attributed to the continued use of a mantra (Omm, Ing, Ahum) is one example.

Wellness, meditation, and relaxation workshops have always made use of music for relaxation, visualization, taking one's mind off of everyday worries, and changing one's level of consciousness. These innovators express that music affords the mind the chance to ease tensions and to flow unattached, which creates a state of mind that allows experience to enter on a different level: internally through the right hemisphere of the brain. This type of experience is not associated with "everyday happenings." It is linked, they explain, to an intrinsic experience that demands that each apply his or her own symbols for meaning, rather than those ordinarily associated with it in life. Music is, in this instance, being used for physical well-being with obvious mental benefits.

Images and symbols representative of health can be applied to music as it is being played. This process can subconsciously "paint" a different perspective than the one presented consciously. Internal processes, through interactions between left and right hemispheres, try to remold the body to conform to the pictures or symbols of health. Elizabeth Philipov, pioneer of music in learning and healing, said it in this way: "With the use, for example, of the image of a flower receiving abundantly the light of the sun, a receptive attitude is suggested. While a heightened awareness is further created with the flow of the music, the identification of the human being with the flower is suggested. The assumed new identity has the suggestive effect of symbolic metamorphosis and can lead to valid inner change" (Philipov, 1979).

You have probably determined by this point that music therapy is not a formal holistic method. Just as holism is on the fringe of allopathy, music therapy borders holism. Music "enhances" many orthodox and unorthodox medical practices, but it has not yet found its place in healing. Since music therapists and the field itself have not yet developed the healing aspects of sound, we propose that interested consumers implement a home enrichment project to take advantage of the healing qualities of music.

Type of Healing

At first we considered music therapy as a natural method. This was because therapists could not prescribe drugs and most do practice some holistic procedures. Clinics, educational seminars, various individual alternative healing methods, self-awareness groups, and modern researchers put music into practice in their own unique versions of well-being and prove its legitimacy. Within these settings music usually plays a secondary role in the overall practice, with its effects being sought to enhance specific awareness exercises or balance the hemispheres of the brain. These methods demonstrate that music therapists are extending the natural methods of music therapy into the laboratory, where computers and other technically sophisticated instruments of modern science are being used scientifically to validate the natural abilities of music as a healing tool.

Music therapists who practice outside of institutional settings and within a private situation work with individuals referred to them. They employ the types of methods discussed earlier as well as innovative measures for home use of music after formal therapy has ended. Many private therapists recommend that clients apply practice measures two to four days each week for relaxation, communication, exercise, and integration. Integration is considered important for maintaining physical, mental, and spiritual well-being in that it involves trained right-left brain processes as well as movement and creativity.

Now let us try to analyze the benefits of the music procedures in relation to the general well-being of any individual. The relaxing procedure aids in easing stress and strain encountered during daily living. One is open to new experiences without feeling the pressures of the old. An alternative energy consumes the body. There is promotion of spiritual insight, a feeling of mental ease, and noticeable physical relaxation.

Fantasizing with music often feeds insights into unknown creative abilities. Right and left hemispherical processes begin to show interaction in life, and beneficial states evolve soon after healees realize they have created their own fantasy. There emerges a belief in control over events and in "personal" power. Fantasy activates mental, spiritual, physical, and emotional growth. Blockages constructed against problems are destroyed, permitting new experiences to change the perceiver literally. The participant's self-controlling factors predominate the old view of reality as primary interrelatedness is encountered with the world at large. The questions provide a new perspective for examining experiences that increase personal awareness. Additionally, people we have worked with on the musical fantasy method profess a greater understanding of those around them as well as increased patience in dealing with common situations.

Happy sounds instill feelings of kindliness toward one's world and faith in the internal unity of self. These tones are essentially faith building in that they reinforce dimensions beyond everyday encounters as one becomes cognizant of states that make up his or her own perception of the world. Expectations that one is "owed" something by life are changed to include a new belief that one is given life to experience. Musical flow bestows faith in a natural harmony that exists in a confusing and seemingly overcomplicated world.

Movement is very important in maintaining physical well-being. Any form of exercise can be performed in conjunction with music. The essential factor is that the body is given the opportunity to move to the rhythm of the sound. A body will naturally choose the pace of exercise to increase harmonious integration between parts. The purpose of any exercise is to breathe deeply, make the heart beat vigorously, and to work up a sweat for at least twenty minutes.

Experts in this field suggest wordless, classical, or natural sounds as most effective for gaining a relaxed, healing state.

Description of Healing Method

We would like to devote this section, which ordinarily describes the healing method, to creating an exercise, expansion, and relaxation program for using music as therapy at home. We will work with both hemispheres of the brain to increase interaction between the two and to aid the growth of the right hemisphere specifically. Physical, mental, and spiritual harmony will be the goal. As wellness and life-style educators, we have a profound respect for the influence of music in promoting healthful changes in one's life, elevating creative abilities, and pinpointing conflicts and inconsistencies. Let us explore the ideas presented earlier in this chapter and apply them to you.

Generally, it is best to choose five pieces of music, each reflecting a different mood. The moods most beneficial for these exercises are relaxing, unfamiliar, happy, a good rhythm or movement, and a thoughty, or "heavy," piece which may or may not contain words. It is best to learn to relax listening to the easiest choice.

The volume should not be too loud or overbearing. In fact, it should be lower than you normally prefer to listen to it. Breathe naturally and contract and relax all muscles. Then, just listen and breathe. The object is to let thoughts, feelings, or pictures that flow into your mind flow out with the music. Halfway through the album or tape you will notice the music sounding louder and all-encompassing. Simultaneously, the thoughts, images, and so on are noticeably absent. At this point you are totally relaxed and your body will tune itself to the music. At the end of the album or tape open your eyes to a more relaxed world and a more balanced physical state.

A second exercise involves playing an unfamiliar piece and observing what thoughts and symbols come to you. Acknowledge these and fantasize about them, expanding the interaction between left and right hemispherical processes. For example, you may have a thought about an overdue car payment. A fantasy can be constructed in which only two payments are left, in which the bank was unusually understanding, or in which someone offered you more money for the car than was paid. Of, if, for instance, a big blue dot appears as a symbol, a fantasy may possibly evolve in which the blue dot is a bubble that carries you to places you have always wanted to visit or that it opens up into a "new world."

To accomplish mood change, one chooses sounds that exemplify this state. Once the choice of music is made, there are several methods helpful in changing your internal state. In a relaxed state you can allow the music to flush out unwanted feelings and allow them to be replaced with the happy pictures created by sound. Let the music carry you. Each time unwanted feelings return, consciously direct them to leave by riding on a joyous note.

Possibly a visualization of better feelings, a particularly appealing scene, or an exciting situation is better suited to your needs. A "real" change has been reported by students practicing the next exercise. Here, we recommend asking thoughts, situations, or feelings to change to happy ones with the music. This is easily accomplished by trying to "picture," in the mind's eye, the opposite thought, situation, or feeling. For example, if you are depressed because your job does not fulfill you, you may visualize the work you wish to do accompanied with how "whole" you feel while creating the job you always wanted.

We have already established that most people have a favorite sound. Further, most favorite sounds will have words. Perhaps the chords are interwoven into an unlikely harmonious combination, or the lyrics present an appealingly idealistic viewpoint. We pointed out that you needed a piece of music to think about, and the next exercise is for that favorite piece, which can merge right and left hemispheres into a harmonious unit as well as expand conscious and subconscious awareness.

Using the music as an intermediary, relax. Concentrate on the piece, allowing your thoughts to expand with the sound. You may "see" the musical score intertwine with the lyrical meaning, the application of those harmonies within your life, how it reflects world feeling, how it releases nature, or how the tones can create a new environment. The more often this is practiced, the more thoughts will emerge. You will know when it is time to choose another piece of music, for all your thoughts will "feel" as if they have formed a composite impression of the music.

Movement and rhythm excite the body. Foot tapping, playing invisible instruments, directing an orchestra, humming, pencil rapping, nodding, finger beating, swaying, and wiggling are often witnessed when music is playing. It is this type of music that is needed for musical exercise. Music is simply the catalyst, a necessary motivation for inactive consumers to exercise those muscles. A number of stretching exercises are relatively simple to perform to the rhythm of music.

Music can be programmed to the desired length of your session. For this reason tapes are often easier to handle so that you do not have to change the record to continue the procedure. Symbols or pictures further enhance the healing qualities of musical therapy. For example, a woman who worked with an unfamiliar piece found it hard to visualize or fantasize. She would look at pictures of great works of art while listening to her music. A gentleman inflicted with arthritis concentrated on the saying "Every day, in every way, I get better and better" while listening to relaxing music. He reported that he felt "tinglings" in his joints and believed that the music gave a "warm flow" to his painful areas. Whenever he was in pain, he recalled the exact sequence of music that released the warm flow.

We do not propose that music can cure all ills. However, it can ease living strains and expand conscious awareness of spirit, mind, and body. Dietary measures must be considered in order to complete a holistic picture, and commitment is also necessary in order to make permanent changes. Music therapy is easily modified to fit individual needs, and the intrinsic benefits show themselves externally in a brief period of time.

Diseases Treated

Music therapy is not a healing method and does not cure dis-ease. However, sound is utilized by music therapists as complementary treatment for the following conditions: behavioral problems, pain, learning disorders, physical disability, geriatric immobility, mental retardation, asthma, emotional disorders, arthritis, rheumatism, cerebral palsy, polio, and autism.

Both orthodox and unorthodox practitioners employ sound in combination with their own therapies. The dis-eases treated, therefore, will vary with the kind of healing method used. Professionals who make use of music include mental health clinicians, psychiatrists, psychologists, sociologists, acupuncturists, nutritionists, Wellness Centers, psychics, dentists, autogenic therapists, and practitioners of massage, yoga, Native American practices, meditation, dream therapy, biofeedback, EST, physical therapy and rehabilitation, nursing, and breathing therapy among others. There may be additional treatments that make use of music, but the ones just listed will employ sound more often than the others.

Duration of Treatment

If you are utilizing music therapy as an adjunct to other treatments, the amount of necessary time will depend upon how long that method is used as well as the "diagnosis" of dis-ease. Those who plan to see a private music therapist will likely attend once a week for one or two hours. Overall length of time is approximately six months to one year. Therapists may also hold group sessions in which one attends a morning session with a number of participants. As with all treatment modalities, the average length of therapy varies with the dis-ease. Most private therapists receive their clients from psychiatrists or mental and social health services. Treatment, in this instance, can last a year or longer. The majority of people that are referred to music therapists within institutionalized settings do not ever "complete" the treatment because it is continually incorporated into the body of programs intended for patients.

It is likely that many Americans use music therapy without defining it as such. Consequently, radios, stereos, and tape players with any number of types of music are heard in cars, from apartments and homes, and on beaches and mountaintops. Using the music method at home, you can decide how long it is needed as well as plan the entire program. It is advisable to try the method for six weeks and evaluate it according to what has been learned about yourself, your world, your relationships with others, and the balancing effect it has had in your life-style. This can be accomplished by recording five broad goals to reach and assessing yourself to see if they are attained at the end of six weeks.

Cost Range

Institutional programs—$12,000 per year (room and board included)
Community centers—(usually continuing or adult education courses)—
$17–$35
Hospitals—free
Mental health centers—free to $40
Private therapists—$7.50–$25 per hour

Personal Responsibilities

Ultimately, you assume responsibility for the healing of dis-ease. Practitioners of music therapy are supplementary providers to other healing modes. Unless you perceive a mental disorder that may be alleviated (other than through relaxation, visualization, and self-examination) by a regime constructed by a music therapist, it is best to secure the necessary materials and proceed on your own at home.

Consumers can learn to benefit from relaxation, visualization, and self-examination in order to balance internal processes, integrate hemispherical processes, create general well-being, and learn about his or her own perception of self. Music exudes an internal faith that replenishes the system. You will have to give credence to this faith externally. All holistic practitioners affirm that efforts to inhibit a natural harmony, growth, and creativity promote dis-ease. On the other hand, belief in yourself and your body's unknown abilities generates energy in that direction. Sound offers experiences and expansion of an infinite number of personal characteristics. Acknowledgment of its abilities strengthens its competencies.

Institutions and therapists associated with them are often locked into one or two types of indirect healing through music and are focused on education. Programs are designed for patients, but they are often not varied enought to absorb the average consumer. In fact, therapists themselves compare these programs with classes in schools. We cannot, therefore, recommend that one attend such a program.

It is more difficult to find natural sounds or tones than it is to find music. This type of "music" may have to be ordered by a favorite music supplier or, for those with recorders, taped by you. While researching this chapter we visited four well-stocked stores to find two meditational albums and one album of whale sounds. Chants were nonexistent. Eastern music is easier to locate than other types, and most of it does not contain words. If you prefer meditational or natural sounds, we have included the names of suppliers in the following section.

Informational Organizations

National Association for Music Therapy, Inc.
PO Box 610
Lawrence, KS 66044

Music Therapy Center
251 West 51st Street
New York, NY 10019

Spectrum Research Institute
231 Emerson Street
Palo Alto, CA 94301

Inner Sound Institute
1572 Beacon Street
Brookline, MA 02416

To locate and/or obtain special music selections, the following will be of help:

Spectrum Research Institute
231 Emerson Street
Palo Alto, CA 94301

Unity Records
PO Box 12
Carte Madera, CA 94925

Consistencies

1. The extensive research on music by Lazanov and Philipov alludes to the advantages of music, tones, and sounds in educating and healing. More recent research indicates that music increases the use of the right hemisphere of the brain, enhancing learning, behavioral changes, and creative expansion. The full implications of these findings for holism are still being explored.

2. Harmony emerges as a naturally integrative approach to spirit, mind, body, and emotions, emphasizing the whole person. Thus, the philosophical concept of harmony in healing may therefore be tied to the use of music by holistic healers as a therapeutic tool in the future.

3. Symbols and visual representations created by listeners provide insight into views that relate to well-being and/or dis-ease. These metaphors of wellness or illness can be employed to rebuild a healthy mental and physical image.

4. Expansion of place or position in the world accompanies a feeling of self-esteem when music therapy is used on populations of emotionally disturbed individuals. Recent research in holism supports the belief that self-esteem is connected with physical and mental well-being. Music therapy, then, can be employed by well populations in order to enhance their ability to experience well-being and improve physical health.

5. The sophisticated technology currently available provides health professionals with an excellent opportunity to expand their field by using music as a fundamental basis for health maintenance and health promotion. The philosophy of holistic healing, along with current research in music, allows for this evolution of contemporary health care.

Inconsistencies

1. The supplemental nature of music therapy exemplifies that it is not employed except in combination with other approaches. It is not, therefore, a complete holistic method.

2. Except when included with other holistic approaches, no mention was made by therapists of dietary importance, counseling, or life-style education and their relationship to health. This fact further illustrates the necessity for rebuilding this field along holistic lines.

3. The majority of therapists are limited to institutions, health centers, prisons, and nursing homes confining their expertise to a select segment of the population rather than serving the entire population. The shortage of music therapists needs to be eradicated before this profession can improve its image within orthodox and holistic health fields.

4. By definition, music therapy neither treats nor heals the spiritual aspects of dis-ease, although it has the potential for accomplishing both. Ancient civilizations used it. Perhaps we should study those uses and attempt to apply them in modern settings.

5. Research by scientists working in this and other fields has only been conducted on behavioral or learning factors enhanced or changed by the use of music. As long as the experts in the field place these boundaries on the method, it will remain dormant.

6. Therapists have done little to advance their field or to incorporate music into distinct adjunctive methods. Although the current areas of music therapy do deserve special attention, therapists need to step forward and make use of their knowledge.

Sources to Read

Alley, Jane M. "Music in the IEP: Therapy Education," *Journal of Music Therapy* 16, no. 3 (1979), pp. 111–27.

Alvin, Juliette. *Music for the Handicapped Child.* London: Oxford University Press, 1965.

Bailey, Phillip. *They Can Make Music.* London: Oxford University Press, 1965.

Bauman, Edward, et al. *The Holistic Health Handbook.* Berkeley, CA: And/Or Press, 1978.

Blair, Lawrence. *Rhythms of Vision.* New York: Warner Books, 1977.

Bloefeld, John. *Mantras: Sacred Words of Power.* New York: Dutton, 1977.

Bonny, Helen, and **Savary, L.** *Music and Your Mind: Listening with a New Consciousness.* New York: Harper and Row, 1973.

Braswell, Charles; dileo Maranto, C., and **deCuir, A.** "A Survey of Clinical Practice in Music Therapy Part I: The Institutions in Which Music

Therapists Work and Personal Data," *Journal of Music Therapy* 16, no 2 (1979), pp. 50–69.

Bricklin, Mark. *The Practical Encyclopedia of Natural Healing.* Emmaus, PA: Rodale Press, 1976.

Bright, Ruth. *Music in Geriatric Care.* New York: St. Martins Press, 1973.

Brydon, Karin A., and **Nugent, W. R.** "Musical Metaphor as a Means of Therapeutic Communication," *Journal of Music Therapy* 16, no. 3 (1979), pp. 49–53.

Feldenkrais, M. *Awareness through Movement.* New York: Harper and Row, 1977.

Gaston, E. T., ed. *Music in Therapy.* New York: Macmillan, 1968.

Halpern, Stephen. *Spectrum Suite: A Record of Meditation Music.* Palo Alto, CA: Spectrum Research Institute, 1977.

Hamel, Peter M. *Through Music to the Self: How to Appreciate and Experience Music Anew,* trans. F. Lemesurier. Boulder, CO: Shambhala Publishers, 1979.

Helene, Corinne. *Beethoven's Nine Symphonies.* Oceanside, CA: New Age Press, 1963.

———. *Color and Music in the New Age.* Oceanside, CA: New Age Press, 1965.

———. *Music: The Keynote of Human Evolution.* Oceanside, CA: New Age Press, 1965.

Iases. *Inter-Dimensional Music.* Corte Madera, CA: Unity Records.

Kaslof, Leslie J. *Wholistic Dimensions in Healing.* Garden City, NY: Doubleday, 1978.

Keyes, Laurel Elizabeth. *Toning: The Creative Power of Voice.* Marina del Rey, CA: De Vorss, 1973.

Liederman, P. C. "Music and Rhythm Group Therapy for Geriatric Patients," *Journal of Music Therapy* 4, no. 4 (1967), pp. 126–27.

Losanov, G. "The Nature and History of the Suggestopedic System of Teaching Foreign Languages and Its Experimental Prospects," *Journal of Suggestology and Suggestopedia* 1 (1975): p. 5–11.

Morena, Joseph J. "Musical Psychodrama: A New Direction in Music Therapy," *Journal of Music Therapy* 4, no. 4 (1967), pp. 34–42.

Oyle, I. *The Healing Mind.* Millbrae, CA: Celestial Arts, 1975.

Philipov, Elizabeth. "Western Approaches to Wholistic Healing," in *Dimensions in Wholistic Healing: New Frontiers in the Treatment of the Whole Person,* ed. Herbert A. Otto and James W. Knight. Chicago: Nelson-Hall, 1979.

Priestly, M. *Music Therapy in Action.* New York: St. Martins Press, 1975.

Reik, Theodore. *The Haunting Melody.* New York: Grove Press, 1960.

Rieger, Jennifer. "Comparisons of Reality Orientation Program for Geriatric Patients, with and without Music," *Journal of Music Therapy* 17, no. 1 (1980), pp. 26–33.

Roskam, Kay. "Music Therapy as an Aid for Increasing Auditory Awareness and Improving Reading Skill," *Journal of Music Therapy* 16, no. 1 (1979), pp. 31–32.

Samuels, Mike, M.D., and **Samuels, N.** *Seeing with the Mind's Eye: The*

History, Techniques and Uses of Visualization. New York: Random House, 1975.

Stebbing, Lionel. *Music: Its Occult Basis and Healing Value.* East Grinstead, Sussex, England: New Knowledge Books, 1974.

Winckel, Fritz. *Music, Sound, and Sensation.* New York: Dover, 1967.

Winston, Shirley Rabb. *Music as the Bridge: Based on Edgar Cayce Readings.* Virginia Beach, VA: ARE Press, 1976.

Zuckerkandl, Victor. *Sound and Symbol.* Princeton, NJ: Princeton University Press, 1969.

CONCLUSION

Critics of conventional health care often characterize the relationship between physician and patient as a major reason why alternative practitioners are sought out and utilized. One of the most basic critiques of conventional physicians is that they have created a system of treatment that is dehumanizing. The presence and cost of sophisticated medical technology, drug treatment, and modern surgical techniques, say the critics, destroys the doctor-patient relationship. These critics give the impression that conventional physicians are often more interested in their social commitments than their patient schedule, as evidenced by the long hours consumers spend in waiting rooms. When reading this literature, one is also given the impression that patients are "conditioned" to forgive their doctors of things they would usually consider unpardonable in normal situations. In other words, physicians are gods and patients cater to their whims no matter how inconvenient.

The clients or former clients of holistic healers we interviewed emphasized the quality of modern health care as a major reason for their shift to holistic health. They felt that in conventional medical practice the consumer had "no control" over his or her health. Generally, the holistic practitioners they visited encouraged them to regain control over both their lives and their health. Others explain that no matter what the field, holistic health was more natural in that fewer technological devices were employed by legitimate holistic healers. To the clients, health was something they could take home with them rather than something that they had to go out and get.

Two other reasons for visiting a holistic practitioner, which we had not seen referred to before but which were paramount in the minds of consumers and the literature on these methods, were that conventional medicine had failed to provide a "cure" for their dis-ease and holistic medicine was actually a principal component of the person's traditional culture.

First and foremost, whether a method is conventional or not, consumers are concerned with whether it works. This reason has both positive and negative consequences. On the positive side, people are not afraid of changing and thereby are less likely to be duped. On the negative side, consumers tend toward an overreliance upon method of cure and become dependent upon the healer, whether his or her orientation is allopathic or homoeopathic. There are many physicians who believe in the self-regulating nature of the body to heal itself but who end up pandering to hypochondriacs by prescribing pills!

The holistic practices we have described in this book possess some common traits, which imply that these methods can work together for the consumer. The philosophy of each field mentions the fact that the technique is employed for the expressed purpose of pinpointing the underlying source of dis-ease, igniting the self-regulating process of the body, and dissolving the basic reason for the dis-ease. What is unique to each field is the history of the founding and the invention of the method. Even here there are similarities, in that the vital force, the life force, Mother Nature, Chi, orgone, or energy centers and essences are referred to as the original focus of the healing process.

Another commonality among all of these holistic modalities is that the legitimate holistic practitioner will subscribe to the belief (and practice) that health should become an intrinsic value of the client. None of the healers were threatened by self-health strategies, health maintenance, or prevention techniques that were being employed by clients on their own. Through body awareness and education the consumer emerges as competent to handle his or her own health on a day-to-day basis. Should a healee require more intensive help from a healer, he or she is prepared to describe symptoms accurately and then to actively participate in the healing strategy. Since practitioners and clients work together to restore and maintain health, healees are enlightened about the multitude of factors that contribute to well-being. In many instances, this knowledge enables the consumer to subvert and/or prevent dis-ease. We are of the opinion that the changes the consumer makes in the area of health could provide the impetus for alterations in other areas.

An impressive characteristic of holistic practitioners is the fact that the "spirit" is within everything and that faith is the fundamental basis for cure, regardless of the specific technique. Since they are a part of the total "makeup" of the universe, spiritual matters affect health and well-being and are not confined to the church or to cultural beliefs. Spirit is akin to life purposes, personal ideals, essential yearnings, and self-fulfillment. "Mind," in this system of beliefs, becomes the vessel through which spirit operates on an everyday basis. A mind can be specialized and focused or imaginative, emotional, or indifferent, intelligent or not. When it comes to the expression of spiritual ideals in practice, the body is the instrument that moves through life taking on and giving off spiritual energy.

These definitions reveal how spirit, mind, and body are interconnected, life-furthering, and creative. Holistic practitioners may make use of many different methods, just as scientific professionals do. The major difference between the two is that holistic healers also possess faith in the belief that the individual can heal him- or herself and that the methods are merely tools used to initiate the natural process of healing. These principles are incorporated into the most frequently mentioned healing strategies used by holistic healers in their educational programs: nutrition, exercise or physical manipulation, stress reduction and/or relaxation, self-care and self-examination, counseling and life-style change, and natural botanicals.

Perhaps it is this common foundation which makes it essential for consumers to approach holistic fields without a questioning attitude, for this branch of health care contains healers who are deceptively claiming the label. From our research we have extracted a number of guidelines to enable consumers to determine if the healer they choose is legitimate. Perhaps the most important point upon which to base your choice is whether or not a practitioner's beliefs, values, and personal characteristics parallel your own. For example, if you are Italian-American, it is unlikely that a Native American practitioner would conform to your beliefs. Likewise, a deeply religious individual may feel comfortable with spiritualism, whereas a "back to earther" may gain a great deal from herbalism. The remainder of the criteria in the following list are self-explanatory.

Criteria for Evaluating a Safe and Reliable Holistic Practitioner

1. Choose a practitioner whose beliefs are similar to your own.

2. Be sure to ask current or previous patients about cost, health strategies they have experienced, and relief (or lack of relief) received from the practitioner.

3. Question the staff about the kinds of methods the practitioner commonly uses.

4. Find out if the practitioner is certified and/or licensed either through formal educational training, extended training, or both.

5. Avoid practitioners who employ persuasive phrases to entice you into accepting a treatment. This includes indirect evidence about a treatment or "smooth talk."

6. Be skeptical about practitioners who will not work with structured physicians or who claim to heal all who come for treatment.

7. Practitioners who do not teach health maintenance practices for home use are not holistic.

8. Practitioners who do not include physical exercise, relaxation, nutrition, and self-examination are not holistic.

9. Ask if the practitioner will outline the responsibilities of healee and healer in writing. If such a contract is not used by the practitioner, ask if he or she objects to one. If so, get a second opinion.

10. Choose a practitioner according to your own definition of the ideal holistic healer.

11. **Only** frauds guarantee results.

Along these lines, there are also some obligations that must be assumed by the consumer, which can enhance any holistic system or treatment and also provide a line of communication between you and your healer. As we have seen in this book, the patient who is involved in his or her health program gains more from the treatment provided by a healer. A patient's compliance with a practitioner's health recommendations can be active or passive. Active consumers integrate health and well-being into their lives, whereas passive consumers merely become acquainted with health.

Consumer Health Responsibilities

1. Familiarize yourself with the field of health you have chosen.
2. Integrate health strategies into your life-style.
3. Read up on an illness, so you are aware of how it manifests itself.
4. Learn to read your body's signals about dis-ease.
5. Approach health with realistic expectations, which include building health one step at a time.
6. Have faith in your body's ability to heal as well as your own control over health and well-being.
7. Cultivate interdependence between you and your health practitioner.
8. Actively reinforce health states in yourself and others.
9. Think of health as an ongoing process.
10. Look for health rather than dis-ease in yourself and in others.

At the conclusion of our research and our writing, we come to a final point. It is the fact that the modern art and science of healing, whether in the allopatic or the holistic camp, was originally based upon a common assumption, the principle of homeostasis. A clearer recognition of the natural self-regulating mechanisms of the body has brought forth a return to holism. Though it is not the same holism that was initiated by Hippocrates, it does seek to return the "force" to modern medicine by merging science with the self-regulating processes of the body. Even though the consumer is likely to be caught between allopathic and holistic forces for some time to come, this common assumption demonstrates that the bridge between them already exists. Although divergent "methods" are clearly the focus of the debate, the natural capability of the body to regulate, adapt, create, and further health is a common interest of both types of practitioners. As the allopathic and holistic fields adapt to change and create new strategies, both sects are being regenerated. This rebirth reflects our own individual concerns for growth. As consumers of both types of health care, we can transfer their faith in us to ourselves so that, in the future, we can create a complementary system supported by all of us.

GLOSSARY

Absent healing—A type of spiritual healing wherein clients mail requests for healing to a group of individuals who pray, imagine, and visualize healing taking place. The meetings are usually scheduled for a specific time and day each week.

Acupressure—A form of acupuncture where needles are replaced by fingertip pressure on the correct loci. The pressure produces an effect that is similar to the use of needles. This technique has also been combined with other healing modalities.

Acupuncture—A traditional Chinese medical system wherein the life force (Chi) of the individual is affected by pressure on acupuncture loci, or points. It is most commonly associated with needles, but in fact, treatment includes massage, acupressure, counseling, relaxation, exercise, and dietary structure.

Alpha waves—Indications on biofeedback devices that denote that one is totally relaxed yet consciously aware. Biofeedback machines record brain waves.

Arndt–Schulz law—This law states that small doses excite reactions, medium doses favor reactions, and large doses dull or stop reactions. It was used by Hahnemann to support the use of the infinitismal dose in homoeopathy.

Association—A list of actors, objects, settings, or words is assembled by dreamers when practicing this dream translation technique. The items are compared with the dreamer's emotional identification with them and their symbolic relevance to the dream.

Astral body—According to psychic healers, this is one of the three centers of psychic energy where the body is perceived by the psychic as emotional "colors." Healers "read" the emotional states of the body by seeing the intensity of colors.

Autogenic therapy—A meditative therapy combining hypnosis and deep relaxation.

Balance—A state of equilibrium in which all portions of the individual are functioning smoothly, adjusting to change properly, exchanging interactions freely, and expanding personal potentials creatively.

Biofeedback—The process by which brain waves are discovered by use of a machine that "feeds" back biological information to the individual. It is often used to train individuals to reach relaxed states.

Body therapy—Adjunctive or supportive methods of massage, manipulation, and finger pressure that removes obstructions from energy channels.

Botanicals—Herbal medicaments that contain natural qualities and are able to "ignite" the self-regulatory processes of the body.

Chi—The ancient Chinese term used by acupuncturists to refer to the life force, life energy, or vital force. The life force is carried through the body along meridians and flows in generative and destructive cycles. Chi is composed of the polar opposites of yin and yang. These forces must be balanced in order for a person to experience health.

Chiropractors—Licensed health professionals who focus upon correcting subluxations in the spine by using reflex adjustments. Holistic chiropractors are also concerned with preventing the recurrence of subluxation through exercise and education.

Creative dreaming—A dream state, much like lucid dreaming, used by inventors, artists, intellectuals, and others as an experimental medium for applying and trying out new ideas before giving them physical form.

Chromotherapy—A naturopathic healing strategy where colors are used to produce beneficial variations in a depleted system, perhaps due to their vibrational quality.

Dick-Read method of natural childbirth—Patterned along the same lines as the Lamaze method, this procedure uses Pavlov's theory of conditioning to prepare parents to deliver the newborn naturally.

Dietitians—Health professionals who specialize in dietetics, the branch of nutritional science concerned with hygiene, and who are responsible for designing special meals for a large number of people. Comparing dietitians with nutritionists becomes meaningless in the field of holistic health, since either can be known as nutritional therapists.

Doctrine of signatures—Used in many traditional medicines for identifying useful botanical substances that are similar to the source of dis-ease. For example, the herb liverleaf is used to treat liver ailments because its leaves resemble the liver.

Dream incubation—A method of dream construction in which the dreamer tries to program a specific dream by concentration, visualization, and association.

Dream therapists—Practitioners who teach that dreams are symbolic pictures of health and dis-ease and that dreams can serve to warn us of physical problems.

Emperir—The name acupuncturists give the active ingredient in herbal remedies. The empirir's aid is called the minister, and the catalyst plant that helps transport the remedy throughout the body is named the ambassador.

Essences—Herbal remedies that have been reduced from the whole plant to an oil. Some feel that these substances are more effective or potent than teas or tonics for affecting the vital force.

Etheric body—The spiritual body that psychic healers claim is responsible for the flow of life energy into the physical body. When imbalances of the life energy occur, dis-ease begins, finally manifesting itself in the physical body.

Family Centered Maternity Care (FCMC)—A combination of professional care, prepared delivery, and shared family experience seeking to bring the comfort of home into the delivery setting.

Generals—A word that is used by homoeopaths to describe physical, mental, and changing symptoms of dis-ease.

Guided imagery—A music therapy technique where the client relaxes to music while the therapist examines feelings, images, or symbols that emerge from the client in an attempt to understand the clients subconscious.

Herbalists—Those practitioners who suggest natural botanicals such as powdered or dried mixtures, oils, ointments, lotions, extracts, teas, or tinctures to affect the vital force.

Holistic health—A health model founded upon the belief that the individual is composed of physical, mental, spiritual, social, environmental, and emotional components. While under the care of a holistic practitioner, the individual must be examined and each part of him or her balanced so that the inherent self-regulating properties of the body can assume their natural role. Holistic health also embraces the policy that the underlying causes of disease must be resolved and that the patient is an active participant in health care.

Holistic health elements—Common treatment elements integrated into many assorted holistic fields are nutrition, exercise, counseling, spiritual awareness, patient education, bodily awareness, relaxation, and life-style change.

Home delivery—A birthing alternative where the child is delivered at home by parents with the support of friends or qualified health professionals. Classes are available to teach breathing, toning, sanitizing, relaxing, birthing processes, and body coordination. This method of birth is not recommended by many physicians, but LeBoyer assistants and nurse-midwives are willing to deliver at home.

Homeostasis—The natural or inherent ability of the body to regulate its functions and processes as well as adapt to change. In holistic health, homeostasis is initiated by balancing physical, mental, spiritual, and, in some cases, emotional, social, and environmental components of the individual.

Homoeopathy—The holistic health system based upon the Law of similia—"like cures like." Founded by Dr. Samuel Hahnemann, homoeopathy ignites the self-healing abilities by prescribing one, infinitismal dose that in gross amounts would create reactions similar to those the patient is experiencing.

"Hot seat"—A common method of dream interpretation carried out in dream groups where participants swap roles with dream characters.

Infinitismal dose—As prescribed by homoeopaths, it is the one correct substance that would affect the vital force and that duplicates the individual's composite of symptoms. The dosage is tested on human beings and is highly diluted so that it initiates homoe-ostasis.

Inner energy—The term used by some meditators to refer to the vital element in the body that is balanced through the use of meditation.

"King's touch"—The "healing touch" of the monarch bestowed upon afflicted subjects on special occasions. The divine touch was attributed with miraculous cures much like those of spiritual healers.

Lamaze—This prepared birthing method consists of utilizing condi-tioned reflexes learned by mother with breathing procedures and the father's aid to deliver a child without the use of modern drugs for anesthesia.

Law of cure—A model used by naturopaths and homoeopaths which assumes that symptoms leave the body in reverse order of their appearance, the most recent symptom leaving the body first with the remainder following successively. The client is said to be experiencing a "healing crisis," which indicates treatment is working.

Law of similars—The natural law proclaimed by Hippocrates that states that dis-ease is cured by application of the like. In homoeopathy, the patient is treated with a remedy that in quantity would produce symptoms like the dis-ease.

Laying on of hands—A technique used by Native American, psychic, and spiritual healers, sometimes known as therapeutic touch or the healing touch. A heatlike energy is released by the healer and often felt by the healee as a mild electrical discharge or warmth.

LeBoyer—An alternative birthing method that welcomes the newborn in a unique manner and can be performed in the hospital or home setting. Delivery is slow and in a quiet room with soft light; the newborn is placed with mother and then given a warm bath to introduce the child to life gradually.

Loci—Loci are points along meridians that correspond to various parts of the body. Acupuncture practitioners contact the life force by applying pressure or employing needles on loci.

Lucid dreaming—Dreams where the dreamer becomes consciously aware of and changes or participates in the contents of dreams.

Meditation—A deeply relaxed state in which one can "let go," or transcend.

Medium—The most frequently reported fraudulent psychic healer who claims to contact the spirits of dead relatives and loved ones in order to solve problems related to dis-ease.

Mental body—In psychic healing, the mental body is composed of thoughts, intuition and memories. According to psychics, the mental body motivates our day-to-day actions within life.

Meridians—The physical pathway by which Chi, the life force, is carried through the body in acupuncture. Meridians map a geography of the body and run from head to toe and side to side.

Mixers—The division within chiropractic that argues for the differential diagnosis and treatment of dis-ease rather than only locating and correcting subluxations. They "mix" a variety of techniques along with spinal realignment.

Moxibustion—The traditional practice of acupuncturists where the dried seed of the mugwort plant is placed on the end of a needle and lit. Practitioners believe that heat and healing energy travel through the needle and into the body.

Music therapy—The profession of adjunctive therapists who feel their services are most effective on behaviors and disabilities within hospitals, clinics, day care facilities, community mental health centers, and prisons. Music is most often integrated into other healing methods.

Native American healing—Healers believe that human beings and the universe are interdependent. In order to maintain harmony or health, healers work with all the energies in nature. When dis-ease occurs, intricate rituals are performed, requiring all members of the tribe to take part.

Native American healing ceremony—Rituals in which Native American healers symbolize man's interrelationship with the natural world. Healing rituals encompass music, dance, song, prayer, and social interaction depicting man's relationship to the whole and the healee's conquering of dis-ease.

Naturopathy—The field of healing founded by Dr. Benjamin Lust, which originally included homoeopathy, herbalism, manipulation, nutrition, psychology, massage, meditation, medical electricity, and hydrotherapy. Naturopaths believe that dis-ease is caused by violations of the natural law of homeostasis, and natural means are best for restoring balance in spirit, mind, and body.

Nurse-midwifery—A specialized health care practitioner who supplies instruction, care, and backup for natural childbirth. Delivering at home or in a hospital, he or she relies upon breathing and pelvic exercises and the body's innate abilities to bring about a birth that is "mother conscious." Although these nurses receive postgraduate training, they are not allowed to practice in most hospitals.

Nutrition—A science concerned with the use of foods for body function.

While diet is the sum total of all the substances consumed, nutrition only includes those substances that nourish or promote growth, maintenance, and repair in the body.

Nutritional or natural food faddists—Those self-styled experts who promote nutrition as a cure of dis-ease with claims of miraculous cures through natural foods, a specific food, supplements, or megavitamin therapy.

Nutritionists—Those scientists and educators who specialize in the problems and processes of nutrition. The distinction between nutritionists and dietitians becomes ambiguous, since both are nutritional therapists.

Particulars—A classification of rare, strange, or peculiar symptoms used by homoeopaths as part of their symptom-gathering diagnosis.

Passive exercise—An integrative technique employed by many body therapists, usually involving rotation and manipulation of the body parts where they are connected to each other.

Physicalists—The scientific camp that believes in only the physical mechanisms of the body to contract and combat dis-ease.

Polarity therapy—A type of health maintenance that focuses upon massaging energy channels, diet, positive thinking, manipulation, and exercise.

Prayer groups—A group of like-minded individuals who use prayer, meditation, visualization, and song to activate the process of spiritual healing.

Psychic healers—Those who rid the body of dis-ease by extraordinary means when there is no medical, psychological, or physical way to explain its disappearance. Psychic healers believe that the body is composed of different centers of subtle energy: the astral body, the etheric body, and the mental body, which can be cleared of obstructions and balanced.

Pulse diagnosis—The traditional method by which acupuncturists diagnose dis-eases of both the past and present by "reading" six pulses on each wrist. These pulses lead the practitioner to one or more of twelve organs that may show energy imbalances.

Reflexology—Known also as zone therapy. Reflexologists massage along certain points or energy zones located on the hands and feet to correct energy imbalances.

Reichian therapy—According to Reich, life energy flows throughout the body, and emotional resistance to problems causes muscular and character "armoring" to take place, which obstructs the life energy. Reichian body therapy and character analysis are the two most common methods used to reduce armoring.

Relaxation—Methods that teach one to release tense muscle and strained emotional states so that the body is able to balance or adjust itself.

Rolfing—Also known as structural integration, Rolfing is designed to realign body segments into vertical position, thereby balancing the body structure.

Shiatsu—A form of massage imported from Japan with an emphasis on attaining balance of vital energies by massaging points located along acupuncture meridians. Healing concentration and sustained pressure are the primary shiatsu techniques.

Spinal manipulation—A term used to describe the adjustment process carried out by chiropractors to correct subluxations and other postoral conditions.

Spiritual healers—Healers who believe they are instruments or vessels for channeling divine power to provide cures. While this branch of healers overlaps the psychic healers, they are distinct from psi healers because they attribute the power to heal to God, Christ, or the Holy Spirit. Spiritual healers claim their treatments are only supplemental to orthodox medicine.

Straights—A division within chiropractic concerned with the location, analysis, and correction of subluxations, which are detrimental to health. Straights attempt to restore the correct energy balance to the body, after which, it is thought, the body will heal itself naturally.

Subluxation—A mechanical lesion in the nervous system or a partly displaced vertebrae.

Suggestopedic learning—A technique that makes use of unconscious activity to aid learning, material is received by audio and visual sensors while the healee simultaneously engages in active learning exercises.

Tonification—The technique by which acupuncturists use needles to stimulate the vital force.

Topdog, underdog—A technique used in dream therapy where one dream symbol or character takes the dominant role while another takes the subordinate one.

Twirled needles—A technique used by acupuncturists to produce increased numbness or pain relief.

Visualization—A relaxation period where the client "pictures" details for scenes or situations which facilitates imagination. This method often accompanies relaxation measures in holistic practices.

Vital force—An intangible energy that is present in individuals, nature, the world around us, and the universe. Some believe it is contained within the body and flows through the channels or centers. Holistic healers initiate homeostasis by way of the vital force. Other names for the vital force are God power, vibrational energy, energy fields, Chi, life force, life energy, creative force, Mother Earth, and energy centers.

Vitalists—The philosophical school of thought that purports that the life force, (or vital force), in addition to physical mechanisms, is involved in preventing dis-ease.

Waking visualization—A dream technique where a dreamer expands the scope of a dream while awake at various intervals, during relaxation, exercise, before napping, while eating, or engaging in other normal activities.

Water purification—A Native American (and naturopathic) practice of using water and/or steam in conjunction with massage to cleanse and purify the healee and to ensure that energy channels flow smoothly.

INDEX